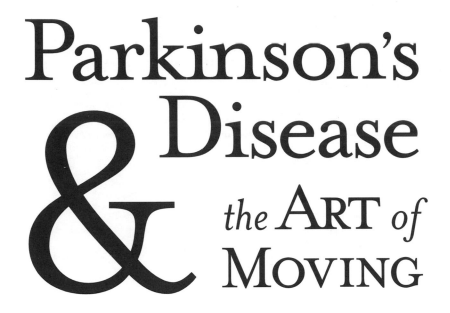

Parkinson's Disease & the ART of MOVING

JOHN ARGUE

NEW HARBINGER PUBLICATIONS, INC.

Publisher's Note

This publication is designed to provide accurate and authoritative information in regard to the subject matter covered. It is sold with the understanding that the publisher is not engaged in rendering psychological, financial, legal, or other professional services. If expert assistance or counseling is needed, the services of a competent professional should be sought.

CONTENTS

Part ll A Dance with the Dragon

TABLE OF EXERCISES

ACKNOWLEDGMENTS

I wish to acknowledge the following friends and colleagues who made this book possible:

Marion Jackson Brucker, for first coming to me with the idea of working with Parkinson's people, and for her steadfast support and encouragement through the years.

My longest running PD class, nicknamed "the board of directors": Marion Brucker, Doug Dickson, M.D., Prof. Owen Chamberlain, Prof. Frank Crawford, Prof. Elizabeth Singer, and Jim Campbell.

My mentor in art-therapy, Eugene B. Sagan, Ph.D.

My Tai-Chi Chuan teachers, Sifu (Master) Kuo Lien-Ying and Simu (Master) Simone Kuo.

My yoga teachers, Mariam Kabeer and Peggy Dey.

All my students in all my classes; what a privilege it has been to serve such courageous people!

NOTE TO THE CAREGIVER

Many of the people who need this book cannot read it. Their eyes cannot follow lines of print reliably. Reading tires them quickly. Many of the people who need to learn the exercises in this book cannot remember a pattern of movement the day after they learned it. They will need someone to read the exercise directions one at a time while they go through them.

The text of the book addresses the person with Parkinson's, but the author and editors understand very well the caregiver's contribution to the patient's success with this program, and we have attempted to design the book with you in mind.

I suggest you read each exercise out loud all the way through to the person you are helping before you ask him or her to begin. Then read one line at a time. When the person has done the action, read the next line. People with Parkinson's need to learn to do things one step at a time; they need to finish each action before they even begin thinking about the next action. The exercises are designed to teach that skill if the person giving directions sticks to this "go slow" approach.

PART 1

BEGINNING

MARION'S STORY

A Personal Experience with Parkinson's Disease

When I began to be troubled by a tremor in my hand in the summer of 1983, I thought it might be stress, since I was in a stressful situation at the time. The tremor came and went, but seemed to occur more frequently as time went on. I began to take piano lessons, with the hope that playing the piano would improve the coordination in my fingers and would be enjoyable as well.

The lessons seemed to help some. I am an artist and left-handed, and it was my left hand that was affected. When my left hand was too shaky, I tried painting with my right hand, and achieved some interesting looseness my painting had not had before. I also liked doing detailed pencil sketches, however, and this intricate work began to be too difficult. One day as I was working on a drawing, I noticed that as I tried to control my hand, my left foot began to shake. This is when I decided to check with my doctor.

He sent me to a neurologist who looked in my eyes, checked all my reflexes, watched me walk, watched me write and draw a spiral with as little wiggle as possible. He watched my foot as I drew, and it trembled, but not much. He said it could be Parkinson's, but he could detect no rigidity, so he just wasn't sure. He prescribed

Artane—two milligrams, three times daily—and told me to observe how it worked and report back in six months, unless I had problems.

I was still holding on to my denial. I *couldn't* have Parkinson's; I wasn't old enough. Parkinson's was crippling; I wasn't crippled.

I didn't know much and didn't yet want to. I joined an exercise club and worked out on exercise machines. Some of the exercises made me shakier, but I figured that was because I wasn't in condition. I swam. That made me feel better—relaxed, supported, smoothly coordinated.

Six months later I returned to the neurologist; I was shakier and showing more definite symptoms. I was diagnosed with Parkinson's disease, and the doctor changed my medication to Sinemet® (generic name: levodopa/carbidopa). The dosage eventually leveled off to three or four tablets of 25/100 (the weakest strength) per day.

After the diagnosis I went into a book store and looked up Parkinson's in a medical book. All that I had been denying to myself was right there, in black and white. Parkinson's disease was a brain disorder that originates in the brain stem and is caused by a slow disintegration of the *substantia nigra* cells; could cause tremor, rigidity, stooped posture, shuffling gait, balance problems, an inability to move, drooling, voice problems, and, occasionally, confusion and memory problems. There were more symptoms, but I had seen enough. I had also seen the word I feared the most: "progressive." So. That was it.

I closed the book, put it on the shelf, and walked out to the car. I felt suddenly dizzy and swallowed the saliva that welled up in my mouth. I just wanted to get home. Fast.

In the months that followed I was alternately frightened about the future of my illness, and confident that I could be one of the lucky ones and suffer only a minor case. After all, I had exercised more than the average person, my coordination had always been pretty good, I ate well, and was generally in good health. I had learned how to cope with stress pretty well and was still working on it with a psychotherapist. I knew I had to experience the fear, cry when I felt I needed to, understand that this was where I was, and with some luck and a lot of support I would be able to get the most out of the rest of my life.

I set up an appointment at the Santa Clara Medical Center (now known as The Parkinson's Institute, in Sunnyvale, California), where I talked to Dr. William Langston, a doctor who was planning to conduct an experiment with a new Parkinson's drug. The interview was exciting, stimulating, frightening. I asked a lot of questions, wanting to appear intelligent and cooperative, like a good candidate for the experiment. The drug, it seemed, had the possibility of boosting the effectiveness of dopaminergics (like Sinemet and its generic equivalents), allowing the patient to take smaller doses and experience fewer side effects. Dr. Langston was hoping that it might also slow down or even stop the destruction of the *substantia nigra* cells. If this turned out to be true, the most frightening word I had read in that short description, "progressive," could be eliminated. If not, I would be no worse off than when I started. I felt I had nothing to lose.

The experiment would be a double-blind study, which meant that half the participants would be on placebos, and no one, not even the doctors, would know which patients were on which drug for two years. Dr. Langston said I would be a good candidate for the experiment, since I had only been on Sinemet for a year and was healthy and in the early stages of the disease. That felt good to me, and I left feeling excited and pleased.

On the way out, I walked by a woman who was sitting in a wheelchair: she was frozen in a skewed, hunched-over posture; her hands were trembling with that distinctive "pill rolling" motion with the fingertips that is typical of Parkinson's; and a thin thread of saliva stretched from her mouth to her lap. I walked by her very fast, jamming my hands in my pockets so my telltale tremble wouldn't show. When I reached my car, my heart was beating fast and irregularly, and my breathing was very shallow. I needed to sit and cry and calm down, blow my nose, and tell myself that I would probably never be as unlucky as that woman, because she had had the disease for years and probably started worse off than me anyway. But I had no time to process my feelings. I needed to drive home from Santa Clara to Berkeley, an hour's drive at best, and it was getting close to rush hour. So I swallowed my fear and set off.

But halfway home I took a wrong exit and found myself on a freeway headed for Hayward, the opposite direction from Berkeley. I found a place to pull off, and this time had my cry, blew my nose, and sighed deeply many times, trying to relax. After about ten minutes I started the car and found my way back on to the right freeway, all the time wishing I had thought to bring someone with me for support.

I think the symbolism of finding my way back on to the right road might have helped my mind begin to focus. The ideas began to flow as I drove along the freeway. I could start my own support group. I could use strategies I had learned from my therapist. I could experiment with methods of exercise and relaxation and see how they worked for me. I could go to meetings of the East Bay Parkinson's

Association, something I had been unwilling—because of my denial—to do. I could talk about the disease to whoever would listen and see what I could find out. I could read Roger Duvoisin's book, *Parkinson's Disease: A Guide for Patient and Family*, which had been recommended to me by Dr. Langston as the most informative and helpful book for the layperson. I would get informed and then add the things I learned from my own experience.

As I drove along on the right road, I began to feel a sense of excitement, a feeling I was on a mission. Perhaps I would get some good from this disease. Perhaps others could too, and perhaps I could help them.

In a hurry now, I took my new ideas back to the neurologist in Berkeley, who had diagnosed my Parkinson's the year before. His lack of enthusiasm made my heart sink. He seemed to feel support groups were silly. He had always been skillful and efficient, but he wanted to treat the symptoms only and never had time to listen to my fears, worries, and speculations. I remembered that when I had asked him what he thought about playing the piano for coordination, he replied, "If you can play with your fingers shaking like that." I didn't need that. I talked it over with my wonderful old family physician, Dr. Bernie Wiegand, and, with his whole-hearted support, I changed doctors.

My new neurologist was as skilled and knowledgeable as the first doctor, but he had a completely different style; he was the kind of doctor who treats the whole patient and not just the symptoms. He liked my idea of a support group and said he had some patients who would be interested in joining one. He even thought he could get me a room in a local hospital where the group could meet. He approved of my volunteering for Dr. Langston's Deprenyl experiment. He also agreed with Dr. Langston that Roger Duvoisin's book was a good book for me to read.

I learned a lot from Duvoisin's book. One percent of all Americans over fifty have Parkinson's disease. It is a disease that is progressive and often frightening in its unpredictability. Though many of its symptoms are controllable with medication, the residual symptoms are always there, reminding the Parkinson's patient that muscles are not responding dependably. The symptoms can override the medications in times of physical and emotional stress, peek through when the effects of the medications wear off sooner than expected, and show up in the morning, before the first pill of the day. The anxiety and stress caused by these constant reminders can exacerbate the symptoms, which in turn will increase the anxiety and stress, and so on. In order to stop this vicious circle, Duvoisin suggested, an informal support group could be helpful, providing a place for sufferers to discuss their symptoms, worries, and fears, and share constructive information. (See *Parkinson's Disease: A Guide for Patient and Family*, Fourth Edition, by Roger C. Duvoisin, M.D., and Jacob Sage, M.D. [Lippincott-Raven Publishers: Philadelphia and New York, 1996.])

But the most important information I got from Duvoisin came from reading two particular paragraphs, which I thought suggested a way to overcome the limitations of this disease. I asked my doctor, my husband, and several other people if Duvoisin was saying what I thought he was saying (I didn't want to be fooled by wishful thinking). Here are the two paragraphs:

> One of the great neurologists of the first quarter of this century, Dr. S. A. Kinnier-Wilson, thought of parkinsonian bradykinesia [literally "slow movement"; that heavy, weary, effortful movement most people with PD know all too well] as a sort of "paralysis of the will." He came to this strangely metaphysical speculation because of the sense of effort and fatigue of which his patients complained. Such speculation, however interesting it might seem, does not help very much. What does "will" really mean? What connection is there between the material structure of the brain and a mental attitude or function such as will?
>
> Other physicians saw patients' complaints that "everything becomes an effort" in another light. They argued that action was being blocked by some dysfunction in the brain. Far from the patients' lacking will power, they were in fact forced to rely on will power to overcome some central blocking or inhibiting effect. One eminent neurologist poetically observed that the patients were "condemned to voluntary movement." It has been noted that in general it is the *automatic acts of daily life that are most affected by bradykinesia, and learned acts less so* [emphasis added]. Hence a severely bradykinetic patient may play the piano very well or execute a tap dance. (From Duvoisin and Sage, Fourth Edition, page 29.)

Perhaps it was the reference to piano playing that tipped me off. I had been making progress, slow but real, with my piano lessons. Was it possible that I could use my artistic studies to counteract the limitations of PD? In the above quotation from Duvoisin's book, the words "will" and "learned" particularly appealed to me. Those words suggested that by studying *conscious* (as opposed to automatic) ways of moving, a Parkinson's patient would be able to function more effectively.

As for the phrase "condemned to," I thought I could change that to "allowed" or "required to use," because, as an artist, I understood about "working within limitations." An analogy might be made to an artist working with a limited palate of colors and wringing everything she possibly can from this limited palate, exploring every possible shade and combination of the colors and shapes she has allowed herself.

A support group could be more than just a discussion group. What I needed was a support group with lessons in conscious movement and voice that would allow me to work within my limitations (Parkinson's disease) while at the same time encouraging me to wring the most out of what I could still do. Such a support group could be like so many art classes I had taken: it could be a structured series of classes that would teach people conscious ways to move and speak. We would be learning a kind of art form—something like acting maybe, with singing and yoga and dance and other things I hadn't thought of yet—to function better within our PD-imposed limitations.

Armed with this insight, I sought out a man who taught acting here in Berkeley. An innovative, avant-garde sort of theater man, John Argue had trained with the same therapists I had studied with: Eugene Benjamin Sagan and Juanita Bradshaw at the Institute for Creative and Artistic Development. I thought John might be the sort of person who would accept my Parkinson's disease as a challenge. It wasn't long before I could see that my intuition was right. John's skills were well adapted to the needs of Parkinson's patients. We began each class with simplified Tai Chi exercises, followed by an assortment of theater games, skills exercises, and vocal and speech training from John's seemingly endless basket of ideas.

After working alone with John for a few years, other people with Parkinson's heard about my excitement with our work, and in the summer of 1985 my solo lessons became John's first Parkinson's Movement and Voice Class. That class is still in session now thirteen years later—John calls it his Board of Directors. He has formed many other classes, some at his studio, some in local hospitals. The program presented in this book grew out of that work.

The class has been a real anchor in my life: the class camaraderie, standing by each other through trips to the hospital for fractures and illnesses, supporting each other after the death of one of our members; after all these years, we still manage to include fun and silliness and wild imagination in our lessons.

And much of this is the result of having such a dedicated teacher. I respect John Argue for his skill, his inventiveness, his compassion, and his faithfulness. Everybody with Parkinson's should have such a teacher. I know my life with this frustrating disease has been so much easier, so much more tolerable, so much less limiting because of my class, my classmates, and my teacher.

    I believe such a program makes sense for everyone with Parkinson's disease. We have a chance here to use creativity, motivation, and work, in addition to the medications available to us, to remain in control of our bodies as much as possible. We can even enjoy the process of learning how to do it.

—Marion Jackson Brucker
August 15, 1999

A Neurologist Explains Parkinson's Disease

Parkinson's disease is a chronic disorder of the brain that impairs a person's ability to move. There is a collection of vital nerve cells in the midbrain that contain a dark pigment called "neuromelanin." In Parkinson's disease, nerve cells within this cluster—called the substantia nigra (black substance)—begin to die for reasons that are not yet clear. One of the major functions of these cells is to produce a neurotransmitter called dopamine; thus, in Parkinson's disease, dopamine levels in the brain become deficient and result in many of the symptoms experienced in the disease. Replacement of the deficient dopamine by levodopa (Sinemet) or by synthetic dopamine-like drugs called dopamine agonists (Permax, Mirapex, Riquip, Parlodel) can provide a dramatic improvement in all the symptoms of Parkinson's disease; yet the disease is progressive, and, over time, the medications tend to lose their efficacy and the symptoms gradually emerge once again.

The symptoms of Parkinson's often develop insidiously, remaining unnoticed until the individual is required to execute certain movements (such as catching a ball, lifting furniture, or playing with children) that overextend the capacity of the stiffened ligaments and muscles. Thus, in addition to the proper use of medications, we must fight this disease by preparing our bodies with a daily exercise routine. Exercise is vitally important for maintaining optimum motor function in individuals with Parkinson's disease. An appropriate exercise routine designed for the individual can compensate for the lack of movement caused by the disease. Stretching is particularly important since this is the best way to regularly achieve maximum range of movement in the joints and ligaments. Another motor function affected by Parkinson's, one that is often neglected in treatment, is voice production. There are numerous muscles involved in producing speech; thus, it is no surprise that vocalization is affected in Parkinson's disease. Voice training (even singing) can do wonders for a person's speech production.

In the following chapters, John Argue provides a comprehensive and unique program of exercises ideally suited for individuals suffering from this disease. The value of these specific exercise routines relates to the underlying brain disorder that is responsible for the symptoms of the disease. In the center of the brain, a network of interconnected nerve cell clusters, called the *basal ganglia*, control many of our movements. Much like a computer, this network appears to store the "complex motor programs" that we use routinely. When we perform a specific motor task, such as picking up a pen, the coordination of all the muscles involved is, in large part, controlled by the basal ganglia. We need only think about picking up the object rather than concentrating on all the intricate muscle contractions involved. These motor actions that we take for granted—walking, writing, eating, dressing, or even smiling—are usually accomplished as if we had an autopilot coordinating the various muscle contractions required to execute these actions.

Individuals with Parkinson' disease gradually lose the automaticity of these movements resulting in symptoms such as reduced arm swing, a tendency to limp or drag one leg, small handwriting (micrographia), loss of facial expression, and a soft monotone voice. A symptom of Parkinson's disease that is nearly always experienced at some time during the course of the disease is slowness of movement. Often this symptom is interpreted as weakness, fatigue, or lack of coordination, but it is actually related to a phenomenon known as *bradykinesia*, which means "slow movement."

The root of all these symptoms can be found in the malfunction of the complex motor programs stored in the basal ganglia. "Automatic" actions do not work well for people with Parkinson's disease.

In *Parkinson's Disease and the Art of Moving*, John Argue introduces a novel approach to exercise for those with this disease. These lessons are based on Mr. Argue's years of experience as an actor and acting teacher as well as his fifteen years experience with groups of individuals with Parkinson's disease. He teaches many of the techniques used in training actors and actresses. To be able to perform, an actor must be in control of his or her body at all times and be able to produce the correct intonation or gesticulation; as Mr. Argue explains, this takes "grace, mindfulness, and completion." Because Parkinson's disease undercuts automatic actions, these techniques are ideal for individuals with this disease: they must learn to move and speak with the same deliberate artfulness required of an actor or actress. They must do almost everything "on purpose" that the rest of us do without thinking.

Ever since I was introduced to John Argue through one of my patients, I have never ceased to marvel at his understanding and devotion to individuals with Parkinson's disease. His exercise groups have been widely acclaimed and are in great demand. Unfortunately, there is only one John Argue; I have often expressed the wish that we could clone him. Therefore, I am delighted that he has recreated his unique approach to exercise in this book, so that I can introduce his techniques to all of my patients.

Remember, getting started is one half of the battle, so read on and experience a new lease on life.

—James W. Tetrud, M.D.
Medical Director
The Parkinson's Institute
Movement Disorders Center
Sunnyvale, California

Parkinson's Disease and the Art of Moving

This program of exercises was developed based on the insight into the underlying nature of Parkinson's disease, which was explained by Dr. James Tetrud in the previous chapter:

> The root of all [Parkinson's] symptoms can be found in the malfunction of the complex motor programs stored in the basal ganglia. "Automatic" actions do not work well for people with Parkinson's.

> In order to deal with your Parkinson's related difficulties, which derive from the loss of automatic movements, you need to learn to move and speak *consciously*. You are "condemned" to conscious actions.

Calisthenics, aerobics, and weightlifting are all important exercises if you wish to lose weight, put on muscle, keep in shape, or build stamina. Those are all legitimate goals, but they are not focused on your Parkinson's problem.

The goal of this program is different: you are aiming at developing a mental ability. Through actions and exercises that you will do with *your body*, you will actually be training *your mind*.

In order to deal with a Parkinson's moment, whether in movement or in speech, you need to learn to go through a conscious procedure:

- You must collect your attention, relax all excitement, and come to an internal stop.

- You need to imagine the action you want to do, and you need to remember or invent the best way to do it.

- Then, with complete and focused attention, you need to perform whatever action you need to do.

- You need to do that action gracefully—that is to say, the easiest way possible that still gets the job done.

- You need to complete that action, and you need to know when it is completed.

- You need to come to an internal stop and focus on the next action.

- You need to remember or invent the best strategy for doing it.

- Then, with complete and focused attention . . . and so forth and so on.

You need to maintain this focused awareness for as long as needed to finish what needs to be done.

Just as these tasks need to be completed one small step at a time, the lessons in this book are made up of short sentences, each directing you to perform one action, usually in a very specific way. Do one instruction at a time; when you finish one, you move on to the next.

The Balinese have a saying: "We have no *Art*, we do *everything* as well as we can." That's where "the *Art* of Moving" comes in. In order to deal with Parkinson's you'll need to learn to do everything as well as you can.

Your overall goal—your strategy for coping with whatever symptoms come along—will be to develop an *artful* way of moving and speaking. An artful action is one that is *graceful*, *mindful*, and *complete*. (These three traits can be remembered by borrowing the initials of a major corporation: "GMC.")

Graceful—You will learn to combine power with ease. When we say, "That athlete (you can substitute dancer, welder, chef) makes it look easy!" we are complimenting that person's grace. Such a person gets the job done with the least amount of fuss or force. In terms of practical skills that you will develop through this program, graceful means:

- taking natural, abdominal, full flowing breaths

- making steady efforts, with gentle persistence and calm repetitions toward success

- fining the easiest, safest way to perform an action

- being able to reverse direction at any moment

For inspiration, watch dancers on TV, or play sports highlights in slow motion.

Workers often appoint a safety committee on their jobs to investigate accidents and prevent their recurrence; you need to become your own safety committee. Learn from every accident or near accident by talking it through in precise detail. You can learn a great deal by actually *repeating* the mistake on purpose, but in slow motion of course. (Actors call this "walking it through"—every fistfight and pratfall must be "walked through" over and over to make it completely safe while it still looks really dangerous.) When you walk through an accident in slow motion, you should do it the "wrong way" on purpose to see exactly *why* it doesn't work. Then you remove any obstacles—a coffee table too close to the chair, a rug on the landing—and figure out a "right way" to do the action safely and gracefully.

Mindful—You will learn to be mindful, intentional, and aware of what you are doing while you are doing it. This is not self-consciousness; it is self-awareness and self-control. In terms of skills you will develop through this program, mindful means:

- relaxed alertness

- your mind is focused inside your body

- receptive attention with peripheral vision and hearing

- mental silence

Complete—To do many things well, you need to do one thing at a time, which means you have to stop trying to do everything at once. Each action has a beginning, a middle, and an end. Come to stillness, then begin. Finish each action, come to stillness, then begin the next. In terms of skills you will develop through this program, complete means:

- having clear movement strategies, which are unhurried and smooth

- performing flowing movements

- finishing your first action before you begin the second

Questions and Answers

Before getting into the specifics of "the Art of Moving," I want to answer some general questions about the relationship between Parkinson's and exercise.

Why do I need to exercise?

Parkinson's disease (PD) is a common disorder of the brain. It develops because of damage to the part of the nervous system that controls movement, posture, and balance. This damage results in a combination of primary symptoms:

- stiffness

- tremor

- slowness and poverty of movement

- difficulty with balance

- difficulty walking

- difficulty speaking

A well-designed exercise program can address all these symptoms with meaningful results. An exercise program can improve the major symptoms, which afflict almost everyone with the disease sooner or later, such as tremor, rigidity, slowness of movement, incomplete range of movement, and uncertain balance. Exercise can also help with the symptoms that appear in some people but not in others, such as gait disturbances, freezing, leg cramps, immobile or "masked" face, decreased blinking, difficulty swallowing, loss of voice power, and speech difficulties. You cannot predict which symptoms may come to you, so it is better to prepare your body to cope with as wide a range of symptoms as possible.

When should I start exercising?

You should start exercising as soon after diagnosis as possible, because PD is a progressive disease. With PD you face an increasing level of difficulty through the rest of your life. Symptoms get worse over time and new symptoms appear. You may be able to delay and prevent the severity of your voice problems, for example, if you have been actively practicing voice exercises in advance. Your worst course of action is to do nothing. For a person with PD, inactivity results in atrophy. The familiar warning holds true: Use it or lose it.

How will this exercise program help me over the long run?

It focuses directly on Parkinson's symptoms. This book presents a series of ten lessons which focus precisely on PD symptoms as comprehensively as possible. Movement exercises are adapted from theater and dance training. Many derive from the principles of Yoga and Tai Chi Chuan, the ancient Chinese exercise art.

It will help you anticipate, prevent, and delay symptoms. These exercises deal with symptoms in advance of their appearance, with an eye to anticipating, delaying, or even preventing symptom emergence. This program can also reduce the harm symptoms can do both to you and to your quality of life. Newly diagnosed people with few symptoms can expect to forestall the appearance of some symptoms, sometimes for years. People with mid-range symptoms can expect to slow their progression and even to reverse the progress of some symptoms with continual exercise. People with advanced symptoms will be able to use the program to a reasonable extent if they take extra precautions for safety and if they give themselves permission to stop working when they tire.

It is paced to your personal needs. Every person with PD proceeds at his or her own pace, and that pace can vary from moment to moment. Your ability to keep pace with exercise directions can turn off without notice. Sometimes your muscles are rigid and unresponsive to your intentions. Sometimes your dyskinesia (involuntary movement, usually the side effect of medication) causes an unexpected movement that can throw you off. Energy loss can come over you suddenly, only to return after a brief respite; sometimes it does not return till your next medication dose comes on. Your unpredictable pace means you need directions that slow down when you slow down and speed up again when you are ready to go again. Since these exercises are broken down action by action, you can work at any pace you are comfortable with.

It is engaging and interesting. Boredom with any exercise program threatens any person's long-term success. This program is engaging and aesthetically pleasing. Think of it as an art form, rather than as calisthenics. Like all art forms, the program offers clear challenges in a safe context, procedural guidance, and a rewarding series of accomplishments over time.

Can I do this program on my own?

You can work alone, but you will probably need a helper part of the time. This book has many exercises, spelled out step-by-step. *It will be difficult for you to read the exercises and focus on what you are doing at the same time.* It will work much better if you get someone else to read the instructions, line by line, at your pace, as you do them.

Now, who could that person be? Your partner, a family member, a personal trainer or a helper, perhaps even another person with PD—you'll probably want to find someone who can read aloud each exercise and, if necessary, attend to your safety. Or you may find that a PD exercise group suits you better. There are many benefits to working with a group.

How can I find a group?

This program is ideally suited to a small group of not more than six people. The benefits to be gained from sharing your path through this incurable illness with a few people in a supportive group cannot be overstated. Your group will share information about how they cope day by day with PD. You will get to know each other and support each other. People who have long-term experience with PD invariably rate the close personal friendships and understanding they get from their exercise groups at the top of their list of support. Your partner or caregiver may also benefit;

by dropping you off at the group, your helpers can take an hour and a half off for themselves.

You may be able to form your own exercise group, which could meet once a week. It would probably be best to hire a movement teacher, someone with a background in teaching theater, dance, yoga, or Tai Chi. Such a person may even have access to a studio where you can conduct the class. The teacher could use this book as the basic lesson plan for your classes.

How do I choose a leader?

If you hire a movement teacher to lead your group, you want someone who provides a living example of the arts they teach. You want a teacher who will do the exercises with you, so you can model your efforts on theirs. Look for a teacher whose voice is beautiful, who moves well, and who is flexible and calm in manner.

Look for a teacher or coach who is *patient* yet *firm*. Avoid teachers who bully and scold. You want that special quality called "tough love."

You also want to avoid people who are too helpful. Although they may seem nice, they are showing their impatience when they leap in and take over. Parkinson's disease is a long row to hoe. You must learn to be patient and firm with yourself; it will help a lot if your teacher is also patient and firm with you. A young and inexperienced person may be better than a person with an armload of credentials, if that young person has the right stuff.

Perhaps a story will help you choose the right person. Thirty years ago, when I had just opened my first acting studio, I sought out Gloria Unti, whose job with the city of San Francisco involved setting up arts classes in community centers. I wanted her guidance about what philosophy should guide my own work at my new studio. I had never seen her before and never saw her again, and I never forgot what she said to me over our cups of coffee.

She had interviewed hundreds and hired dozens of teachers of painting, dance, drama, pottery, music, and any other art form you care to mention. This is what she said: "There are teachers, and there are artists; and then, there are teachers of arts, and *that's* a different breed of cat."

You want to find that different breed of cat, whatever their credentials. You'll know them when you work with them a week or two. You will feel protected, inspired, and challenged; you will be eager to return to class each week. At the same time, you should feel a bit of a thrill, a bit of stage fright, about what you may be asked to do. But you'll do it.

It's worth it to fire a few of the other sort in order to find a real teacher of arts.

I already have some symptoms that limit me. Will I be able to do this program?

These exercises were developed over fifteen years of weekly classes with five different groups. Students stayed with the program for years, some as little as two years, many as long as ten, and one student for fifteen years (Marion Brucker, who wrote the story-introduction, and whose inspiration has contributed so much to this program). The severity of the symptoms has ranged from mild to advanced. In other words, the program has been field-tested, and I've found that, using reasonable caution, these exercises are safe for people dealing with the entire range of limitations that result from PD.

Will this program be expensive?

No special equipment is required; only a few easily obtained items are needed. Your program can be done at home, or at a public space if you work in a group. Hospitals will often make their meeting rooms available for support groups. Senior centers and churches also have spaces that could work. If you find a teacher for your group, the teacher may have a yoga or dance studio where you can meet. You will need to work out your fees with your teacher. Six people in the group can spread the cost of the class around so that your expense is reasonable.

Will this program take a lot of time?

If you work alone with a paid personal trainer, budget one meeting a week for one hour. Group time should be one meeting a week for one and a half hours.

In addition, you will need to use at least one hour every day to do some focused physical activity. Many couples find a budget of one hour a day for physical activity very reasonable. If you have a paid attendant in your home, you may want to use an hour of their time for your home exercise program.

You may want to repeat your lesson on your own every day. Or you may prefer to vary your activities, do your lesson every other day, and get out to do some swimming, golfing, gardening, or walking on the odd days. This program encourages an extension of the skills and aesthetic principles you learn into other life activities, like sports or the arts.

You may manage by yourself just fine, but many people find that exercise hours happen more reliably if you invite someone to accompany you—it could be a friend, a classmate, your partner, a child or grandchild, or somebody new to PD.

Will I fit in with a group? If I'm already getting into mid-range or advanced symptoms, won't I be a burden and hold everyone back?

This program adapts well to the differing abilities of members of a group. Lessons progress from easy and safe toward difficult and challenging, building a coherent hierarchy of skills and abilities. Each lesson has a built-in progression from a beginner's limits toward increasing ability. Therefore, your group participation can be continuous even in times of reduced functioning.

Safety must be your primary consideration. Challenge must be the secondary. Each person must proceed at a pace that guarantees safety, while at the same time taking on enough challenges to make progress.

Here's how this works in one of my classes. The class has been going on at the hospital for almost three years. Eileen has been in the class since its beginning and almost never misses. She has very advanced PD and must take a great deal of medicine to move at all; her dyskinesia can cause her to flail and twist in unexpected directions and more or less continuously. She does all the exercises with those extra jerky movements. She has improved tremendously over the years, partly due to advanced medical procedures, partly due her determination to keep up her exercises. She no longer brings a walker and gave up her cane as well.

She stands in the circle with the others. What she can do she does, in her own way. When her meds go off suddenly, as they do sometimes, we help her sit, fetch her meds, and go on with our exercises. When she can speak again, she entertains us with Irish proverbs and witticisms as she sits there. When she can move, she rejoins the circle.

Donald has been in the class for two years and has a talent for movement. He can do one of the more difficult exercises, *Stand on One Foot*, with his free foot in the air for a full minute, sometimes longer. During that minute, his classmates raise their free foot perhaps six times, hold it for a bit, then gracefully set the foot back to the ground.

One member, Eduardo, is quite an elderly gentleman; during *Stand on One Foot* he braces himself on the back of a chair, lifts his free foot an inch from the ground, and sometimes bounces a bit on the leg he is standing on.

Roger just joined the class two weeks ago. He is given special attention during the sitting warm-ups, and then continues to do the sitting exercises when the class is doing more advanced work. He watches what they do while he does the sitting stretches, and he learns what he can. When he wants to try the new movement, I tell the class to follow Donald for a few minutes while I coach Roger through his first couple of tries. If the movement is too advanced, I teach him the precursory movement that he can do safely. For *Stand on One Leg*, that would be "lift your knee up off the ground while sitting."

Differences enrich us all. Different levels of ability in a class can be accommodated fairly well if

- each person competes only with himself

- each person roots for every other person

- each person takes responsibility to work within his or her personal limits

- everybody looks out for everybody else

- the teacher responds gracefully to a constantly changing situation

Gradually everybody will get a taste for the flowing evolution of each class period. Classes become a play we make up on the spot: an actor-training studio where we do the best we can with what we have and have as much fun as possible doing it. There are no small parts, only small actors; no stars, because we are all superstars. We complain all the time; that's part of the fun.

When is the best time to exercise?

Your workout needs to be done daily (or every other day if you choose another physical activity on alternate days) to have the most beneficial effect. Each day's work will expand your limits. Each day you will stretch just a tiny bit farther, sustain an effort a tiny bit longer, maintain your balance just that much more gracefully. All practitioners of the arts know this, and the successful ones do a daily routine, rain or shine.

A daily routine is not easy for the person with PD. The rain seems to rain harder and more often on those with this baffling disease. You cannot predict how much energy will be available, or whether the medications will be working well or seeming not to work at all. Then there are still the responsibilities of the rest of your life—to your family, to your work, to your friends. How are you to manage?

The hardest part is beginning. Once you start on your way, the work quickly becomes easier. My grandfather had a saying, "It's like getting olives out of a jar; after the first one, the rest come easy."

There are ways to make beginning easier. Choose a certain space in your house where you'll do the workout. Set that space aside as your special workout place. Make it as comfortable and inviting and useful as it can possibly be. Place everything you need right there where you can find it, and leave it there. Put this book there with a bookstand to hold it open to your place. Put your supply of tennis balls, your sturdy chair, and perhaps a glass of water and a box of tissues there. Have a timer there, if you like timers; or put a music player there to play your favorite tapes or CDs. Then time your workout period to the tape, or to an hour of morning radio (television is too distracting!).

Choose a regular time. Most people with PD say they function best in the morning hours. You may think it best to choose first thing in the morning. You need to find what works for you. Carl Simmons has always enjoyed the dawn hours best. He likes to get up at least an hour before his wife wakes up, slip into his loose workout clothes, and take a first cup of tea with him to the back bedroom. He likes to face toward the east and be looking out the window for the first glimmer of the sunrise. He takes a few sips of tea, says a gratitude prayer, and then begins the workout. Once he has begun, "the rest comes easy." Carl has even devised a clever way to time himself. When he hears his wife's alarm go off at the other end of the house, he knows his hour is just about done. When he hears her shower running, he can do his voice exercises as loud as he wants without disturbing anybody.

There are many ways to make your exercise time work. Alice and Marianne meet at Alice's house and do their exercises together: first Alice reads the exercise while Marianne does them, then Marianne reads for Alice. Miguel's wife does the workout with him because otherwise he will doze off; she says it helps to keep her fit. Wilson has a hired attendant who will read through the directions. Find what works for you and stick to it.

How can I keep myself motivated?

Set *achievable* goals for your workout. Don't ask yourself to do too much. Decide ahead of time to work for an hour, and at the end of the hour, stop! Decide ahead of time to do just the first half of the sitting exercises, and when you get to that place in the book, stop. If you still have more time in your hour, go back to the beginning and do the first half of the sitting exercises again. Do them more slowly this time, relax and enjoy them.

This is especially true for you if you know yourself to be an overachiever. If you have always been somewhat driven and have never been satisfied with any job no matter how well done, you will need to train yourself to set achievable goals—goals that are much less than your first impulse would suggest.

Fred Wilson was quite a successful real estate man and did not know the meaning of time off. He had grown up plowing with a mule in Missouri and flew seaplanes for unbelievably long hours throughout the Pacific islands during the war. His sense of humor ran to the ruefully realistic; he would readily admit to a "terminal case of the American work ethic." His approach to the gentlest exercises was to grab them with both hands and throttle the life out of them.

When Parkinson's forced him to slow down, he was too much of a realist to resent it. "That's the hand I've been dealt," he would say, "and that's the hand I will play." He tried to stop pushing himself so hard, but the habits of a lifetime are hard to break. "So," he said, "I sat myself down and gave myself a good talking to." He bought a mat to do his workout at his office, trained himself to loosen his tie in the middle of the day, scheduled his exercise times in his appointment calendar, and had his secretary hold all calls. After a few years he arranged an early retirement for himself, sold the company, and moved to the country. Strangely enough, retirement seemed to reduce his Parkinson's symptoms! He says that learning to relax probably added another ten years to his life.

Don't defeat yourself by working too hard. The danger with trying too hard and doing too much, even if you can force yourself to finish, is that the experience is so uncomfortable that you feel only a mental satisfaction in having defeated your lazy body once again. If you make the exercise grueling, you may develop an aversion to it. It may become harder and harder to make yourself begin.

It's much better to set an achievable goal, one that gives your body just the right amount of effort. Then, at the end of your workout, your body feels refreshed and pleasantly stretched out. You have a double satisfaction: your mind has stuck to the achievable goal and your body feels well taken care of. You will be that much more likely to come back the next day if you can anticipate another "double satisfaction"!

Reward yourself. Any habit, healthy or unhealthy, maintains itself through a pattern of intrinsic and extrinsic rewards. The intrinsic rewards of exercise may be increased competence, a loose and comfortable body, and the mental satisfaction of setting a goal and achieving it. But most of us also have an interior part of us that resists doing *anything* that somebody (even ourselves) says we *ought* to do. Extrinsic rewards can be very helpful in keeping that interior part of us showing up for the workout hour.

Dwight just loved musical comedy. He could sing every song from *South Pacific* word for word. He had a small, precious collection of records of Rogers and Hammerstein's greatest hits, but his wife just didn't care for them, especially after the two hundredth time he put them on. Peace was restored to their home with a trade: first the workout, then the record. Their grown children found out about this wonderful arrangement, and you can guess what Dwight got for Christmas: *more* records (and a set of headphones). Reward yourself for your workout achievements. Think up some special treat—something that's not illegal, immoral, or fattening—that can overcome the resistance of that inner foot-dragger.

Some folks find it very difficult to come up with good ideas for rewards. Propose this as a topic at your Parkinson's support group, and watch the fun. People are often much better at making up rewards for others than they are at thinking up rewards for themselves!

Gina was the kind of person that people call a good listener. During a discussion of rewards, the talk turned to things people had loved to do as children—hobbies and crafts and sports and games. Gina didn't say much at the time, but the very next meeting she showed up with a treasure trove: a model airplane, jacks, a paint by numbers kit, a hand loom with enough yarn for four coasters, and several other goodies. She had picked up everything from the local Goodwill and spent less than ten dollars for the whole shopping spree. She played fairy godmother and passed out her gifts. "Now these are for after your exercise," she said sweetly. People laughed and kidded a lot, but of course they were touched. The point was made: extrinsic rewards can help to build the healthy habit of daily workouts.

Social support can add another strong motivation for staying with a program of daily workouts. It is one of the wonderful mysteries about people: some folks who just can't make themselves do any exercise for their own benefit will turn out regular as clockwork to help somebody else. That's what worked for George.

George read voraciously, sometimes forgetting even to eat, much less exercise. He did manage to attend a weekly support group—perhaps only to tell everybody the great things he was reading—but could never remember to do any workout at home.

In the same group was another man, named Louis. George became worried about Louis's welfare when a combination of PD and a bit of bad luck lowered Louis's spirits. Louis had to give up driving after a minor but scary accident. He put the car away for good. When George found out he volunteered to drive Louis to their weekly support group. Soon George signed them both up for a seniors swimming session at the YMCA. It was a water aerobics class designed for people with heart conditions, so the pool was outfitted with good safety devices. Louis was able to "keep on keeping on" with George's encouragement. And, small wonder, George improved even more!

Make your workouts inviting, achievable, challenging, and rewarding. Think of exercise as serious play; that is to say, think of those movements as an art form. The satisfactions you feel will bring you back the next day ready and willing.

Forgive yourself. Don't be too hard on yourself. Try not to build up an "exercise debt" because you were not able to do your planned workout on any particular day. The burden of guilt may make you resentful and sulky, so just turn that debt loose. Start each day with a clean slate by forgiving yourself for not doing enough the day before. Do for today what you can for today. Forgive yourself, begin again. As the poet Rilke said, "Always be beginning."

What equipment will I need?

You'll need a few simple things:

- a carpeted space clear of all furniture and about as big as a queen-size bed (if you need them, install some grab bars in a few places)

- a sturdy chair with arms

- a small supply of tennis balls, six should do

- an exercise mat if your knees are tender

- a few cushions; bed pillows probably won't do

- a few texts for voice practice: children's books, poems, some famous passages of prose, devotional literature—almost anything will do that is interesting enough to spend some time with

You may want to read through these questions and answers again in a few weeks or months. The answers may make more sense after you've worked your way through some of the lessons. Now it's time to learn the program.

THE LESSON PLAN

The program presented in this book teaches people how to prepare for and overcome many of the difficulties of Parkinson's disease. There are ten lessons. All the lessons are interwoven so that precursory skills learned in earlier lessons will fit together with advanced skills learned later in the series. The whole set of lessons makes a dance: a choreography of movements strung together to be beautiful and meaningful. In this sense the full exercise program resembles Tai Chi Chuan, which teaches the ancient art of boxing with an intricate set of movements done in slow motion. But in this program the opponent is not an imaginary boxer, but the disease itself, in all its complexity, variety, unpredictability, and stubbornness. If Parkinson's disease can be thought of as a dragon, then this choreography may be called "A Dance with the Dragon."

Learn the Lessons One at a Time

This is a graduated series. Each lesson depends on the lessons that precede it. You will need the skills you learn in Lesson 3, "Floor Exercises," when you work through Lesson 4, "On Hands and Knees." You need to have worked with the standing exercises in Lessons 6 through 9 for several months before it makes sense to begin the more complex skills in Lesson 10, "Balance and Recovery."

Each lesson will need at least four weeks of repetition to make enough difference in your strength and flexiblility to qualify you for the next lesson's challenges. Patience pays, both in safety and in refinement. Stick with the old lesson, don't insist on something new. Most people old enough to have Parkinson's are also old enough to know that novelty is a highly overrated quality. Start from the beginning, Lesson 1, and gradually make your way through to Lesson 10.

During the first two months, do Lesson 1, "Sitting Exercises," and Lesson 2, "Voice and Speech Exercises." Throughout the entire program, Lesson 1, "Sitting Exercises," should be done at the beginning of every exercise period as a warm-up. Lesson 2, "Voice and Speech Exercises," should be done at the end of every session as a cooldown exercise.

In each exercise session, you should allot one quarter of the time for warm-up, then one half for new material, and the final quarter for cooldown. In a one hour workout, you would warm up with fifteen minutes of sitting exercises, then move on to thirty minutes of new material, and then cool down with fifteen minutes voice work. In a 90-minute class, the ratio would be 20/50/20.

Warm-ups and cooldowns are important! They insure your safety by focusing your attention and mobilizing your resources. Do them!

During your third month, do Lesson 1 as a warm-up, Lesson 3, "Floor Exercises," as your new material, and finish with Lesson 2, "Voice and Speech Exercises."

During your fourth month, do Lesson 1 as a warm-up, then Lesson 4 "On Hands and Knees," and then cool down with Lesson 2.

In the fourth week of the fourth month, do Lessons 1, 3, 4, and 2, in that order, as a review.

During the fifth month, begin with Lesson 1 as a warm-up, then Lesson 5 "Leg Stretches," as your new material, and cool down with Lesson 2.

In the fourth week of the fifth month, do Lessons 1, 3, 4, 5, and 2, in that order, as a review and as a test of your increasing stamina and agility.

Continue this pattern through the tenth month, when the new material will be Lesson 10, "Freezing, Turning, and Walking."

In the review week after Lesson 10 your exercise session will include all the exercises, in order, from beginning to the end: Lesson 1, 3, 4, 5, 6, 7, 8, 9, 10, 2.

A Month-by-Month Lesson Plan

(Remember, these are only recommended amounts of time. Don't start a new lesson until you are comfortable with the moves in the previous lesson.)

Month	Lesson Order	Review Week Order
1	1, 2	1, 2
2	1, 2	1, 2
3	1, 3, 2	1, 3, 2
4	1, 4, 2	1, 3, 4, 2
5	1, 5, 2	1, 3, 4, 5, 2
6	1, 6, 2	1, 3, 4, 5, 6, 2
7	1, 7, 2	1, 3, 4, 5, 6, 7, 2
8	1, 8, 2	1, 3, 4, 5, 6, 7, 8, 2
9	1, 9, 2	1, 3, 4, 5, 6, 7, 8, 9, 2
10	1, 10, 2	1, 3, 4, 5, 6, 7, 8, 9, 10, 2

Then go back to the beginning and learn the whole set over again. Take just as much time as before. Now that you know the end, the beginning will have all kinds of new meaning and subtlety, and you will understand things so much better. You will be amazed at how easily you can do a movement that was incredibly difficult the first time you learned it.

You may want to extend some movements, change the pace a little, take time to explore your limits, figure some way to change things just a little to see what will happen.

The last session in every month will be a review session in which you do all the exercises you have learned up to that point in one flowing sequence. During review sessions, you do not need to do the full number of repetitions of each exercise: once or twice for each movement will be enough.

At least once a month do the whole set, the full-length "Dance with a Dragon," from beginning to end. (In the early months, do only as much as you have learned so far.) Figure out a way to ease up here or save your energy there, flow from this movement right into the next movement without resting, or slow things down when you need to. Be graceful; be mindful; complete each move, then go on to the next. Celebrate the entire dance.

Dance the Whole Sequence

The person reading the exercises aloud will need to read the name of each exercise and give one or two directions to remind you how to begin. You will probably remember how to complete the exercise without the directions being read aloud to you. Or you may need to be prompted. Reader and exerciser will need to adjust to each other as they go along. After getting used to each other, you will find this is like improvising music together: you, your classmates, and your teacher each contribute your part to the whole, making your own "Dance with the Dragon."

You should try to go from one exercise directly into the next in a smooth flowing transition. Keep your attention concentrated on what you are doing; don't let yourself be distracted. You want to make the whole "Dance with the Dragon" move along with grace, mindfulness, and completion. You want to make this a kind of serious fun.

Always balance challenge with safety. Do the exercises with only the forcefulness that you know is appropriate for you. Another student in your class may be able to do a deeper stretch, hold a strength pose longer than you can, or repeat a movement three times while you are doing the same movement only once. Cheer that person on, but don't let competition lead you into inappropriate risk-taking.

There was a rather magical group working in California in the early 1970s called New Games. Their work involved inventing non-competitive playground games that could include everybody—young, old, able, and disabled, every kind of person who would show up. Their motto, emblazoned on T-shirts that are treasured to this day, was "Play hard, Play fair, Nobody hurt." Let that be your motto during the review sessions.

And Then What?

After you have gone through the entire ten lessons the second time—we're talking somewhere between eighteen and twenty-four months now—you will wonder what to do next. An old joke is instructive:

A very serious young man went to the wise man and asked, "Honorable sir, I know the world rests on the back of an elephant. What does the elephant stand on?" The wise man replied, "There is another elephant." "Ahhh!" said the young man. "And what does that elephant stand on?" And the wise man leaned close and whispered, "There are elephants all the way down!"

In other words, go back to the beginning. Unless they find a cure for PD, you will need to continue exercising for the rest of your life.

Always be beginning.

Think of Parkinson's disease as a dragon. In the old stories, a dragon brings danger, but also hides some rich treasure. If you succeed in your contest with the dragon, you get the treasure. These exercises will give you the means to battle the dragon. The rest is up to you.

May you succeed and win your reward.

PART II

A DANCE WITH THE DRAGON

LESSON 1

. . . .

SITTING EXERCISES (THE WARM-UP)

You begin your work with sitting exercises. Even if you are already in good shape and confident in your ability to do more difficult exercises from the get-go, you should start from the beginning. Start safely and slowly: you shouldn't take any risks until you know exactly how physically ready you are and how your medication responds to exercises. You insure your safety by working in a sitting position first.

Always warm up gradually, with a steady pressure on your physical system to wake it up and get it into gear. It is strongly recommended that you begin every exercise session with these sitting exercises, even after you have completed all the lessons in this book. Remember Rilke's words: "Always be beginning." Professionals in sports and the arts always begin work at the beginning, starting every practice session with the fundamentals.

Remember that this exercise program focuses on **gracefulness,** not vigorous assault; **mindfulness,** not forcefulness; and **completion,** not routine repetitions.

In this lesson you will learn four key ideas. First you will work with a tennis ball to massage and sensitize the soles of your feet and then the knuckles of your hands. You will consider the idea that exercises should "**hurt good**" when they are done with the proper vigor. Then you will learn three spine stretches that will loosen up the whole length of your spine. During these spine exercises you will learn to pay attention to "**kinesthesia**" and "**full tidal breathing**" during your workouts. You will finish off your spine stretches with a playful *Groaner's Yoga,* which will introduce you to the important concept of "**relaxation combined with effort**."

These exercises are all done sitting down, where you will be safe from the possibility of a fall. You'll need a sturdy chair with strong arms and not too much padding. If you are in a wheelchair and that's where you feel most secure, be sure the wheels are locked and the footrests turned out of the way or removed. If you are sure you will not slip off to the side, a strong chair without arms will do. If you are already fairly limber and secure in your balance, try working on a stool with a pad- ded top. Put safety first and choose what works best for you.

You'll need a small supply of tennis balls, about six. You can buy new, of course, but remember that tennis players almost always have a supply of used balls they will be happy to give away. It's a nice way to do a little recycling.

You need to warm up gradually. Professional actors, dancers, and singers always come to the theater early and do warm-up exercises. They know that a muscle can be damaged by a sudden leap into action and that a voice needs to open up gradually to avoid strain. Always start your exercise session gently, then increase the effort as you proceed. This quiet sitting exercise is a good way to begin.

Foot Warm-up

Balance starts on the bottom of your feet. This exercise will massage the bot- toms of your feet, stretching and relaxing tight muscles. Your ankles will loosen up a bit also. This will help you become more conscious of your feet. Try to picture in your mind the way the bones, muscles, and tendons fit together. Wasn't it Michelangelo who said that the most marvelous piece of machinery in nature was the human foot?

EXERCISE 1.1
Ball Under Foot

- Remove your shoes.
- Sit forward on the edge of your chair.
- Place a tennis ball under your foot. (See figure 1.1.)
- Press down on the ball till it "hurts good."
- Roll the ball forward and back under your foot.
- (If it doesn't hurt good enough to suit you, lean forward with your hands on your thigh to increase the pressure.)
- Keep this up for two to five minutes.
- Notice how your ankle starts to loosen up.
- Take your foot off the ball.
- Place your foot gently on the floor.
- Feel the floor with the sole of your foot just as you would feel a table top with the palm of your hand.
- Repeat the exercise with the ball under the other foot.

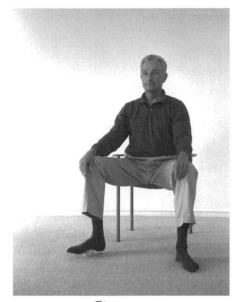

Figure 1.1

It's best to do the *Ball Under Foot* exercise on a carpet. You'll be rolling the ball back and forth with your feet, and on a bare floor, the tennis ball has a tendency to slide out from under your foot. If a carpeted floor is not available, use a yoga mat or a sleeping mat (available at camping supply stores) with a non-slippery surface. You can also make do with a blanket folded on the floor at your feet.

One more suggestion: if you lose a ball, don't bother to chase after it, just let it roll away. You have a supply of six, so just put down another one and continue. Wait till you run out to pick up stray balls, then you can pick them up all at once. Making a quick dive after a lost ball can land you on your nose if you have balance problems. It's probably a good idea to practice letting things go when you drop them; things can be replaced, a broken nose can be expensive.

Ball Under Foot works well if you have circulation problems in your foot. If you remove your socks, you might notice that the blue coloration in your ankle before the exercise changes to a healthier color as the exercise helps push blood up from your feet.

Keep a tennis ball near your favorite chair and do this foot exercise from time to time as you read or watch television.

Hurts Good

Now let's take up the first important idea. Concentrate on the pressure under your foot. Notice how the sensation of comfort and the sensation of pain mix together; we call that mixture "hurts good."

Perhaps you have already guessed what I mean by "hurts good." You may remember a time when people have massaged your tired shoulders and they squeeze a sore muscle and you say "Owwww!" And they say, "I'm sorry! Do you want me to stop?" And you say, "Oh, no, do it some more! It hurts so good!"

That "hurts good" feeling is important in many of your exercises. I recommend that you develop a taste for it! And don't be afraid to make that "Owww!" sound. I always know a class is going well when people feel free to sound off with a chorus of hearty grunts and groans. (Those grunts and groans are good for your voice, too!)

Hand Warm-up

Next come some hand exercises. You will be focusing all your attention on the inner workings of your hands. (You don't need to be too solemn about "focusing all your attention"; during classes you can use both foot and hand warm-up time to chat with folks and catch up on how they are getting along. Just don't get so interested in listening or talking that you stop doing the exercise!)

EXERCISE 1.2
Tennis Ball Stretches

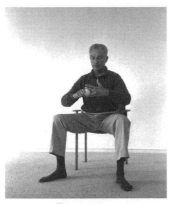

Figure 1.2a

- Take a tennis ball into your hands.
- Hold the ball firmly in one hand.
- Press the ball into the "V" space between each pair of fingers on the other hand. (See figure 1.2a.)
- Press the ball between your first and middle fingers.
- Between your middle and ring fingers.
- Between your ring and little fingers.
- Keep each pair of fingers level with each other; don't let one or the other bend down toward your palm.

- Move right along through both hands.
- Do it again with both "V" fingers *curved* around the ball. (A former baseball pitcher told us this was called a "fork ball.")
- Do this for two to five minutes.
- Next, curve your fingers and widen each hand like a catcher's mitt, or as if you wanted to pick up a soccer ball with one hand. (See figure 1.2b.)
- Widen each hand across the broad part of your palm.

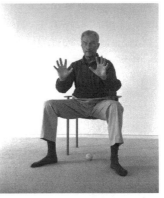

Figure 1.2b

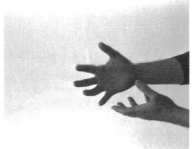

Figure 1.2c

- Relax your wrists.
- Spread your hands wide; keep them loose, not stiff. (See figure 1.2c.)
- Look at each hand carefully; make sure every finger is curved, make sure every "V" between your fingers is open.
- Hold your stretched-open hands for two minutes, down and out to your sides.

Small motor movements in the hands get tangled as a result of PD. Handling a knife and fork, opening pill bottles, selecting a tiny pill from a small heap of pills: these tasks can be tiresome and frustrating. Handwriting often becomes shaky and difficult to decipher; it may even dwindle into the tiny henscratch called micrographia. And if you are one of those gifted people who have written letters to friends and family all your life, what a loss you feel when your handwriting becomes unreadable!

Pamela Barker had trouble with small movements in her hands. She is a courtly lady of eighty-two with a sprightly sense of humor and the amazing ability to touch her toes with her legs straight. We teased her that she was only pretending to be elderly and that she must have dyed her hair gray. She had withdrawn from her much loved bridge club because she could no longer hold her cards properly. After working with the *Tennis Ball Stretches* exercise for a few weeks, her hands improved enough to hold cards again. She was delighted.

Hand exercises can improve the health and functioning of your hands. You can improve your circulation to make your hands feel warmer. You can soften stiff joints and reduce arthritic pain. You could even learn or re-learn typewriting and compose your letters with a word processor or a computer. Just don't give up! Never give up!

Hand Dance with Tennis Ball

You may be able, as you learn the mindfulness techniques in this book, to bring a tremor to rest while you focus your thought into your hand. This next exercise begins your anti-tremor work. Before you begin, let me remind you, if you drop one of your balls, just let it go. Pick up another ball from your supply of six and go on with the exercise. It's more efficient to wait and collect all the lost balls at the end of the exercise period.

EXERCISE 1.3
The Basket

· Make a loose basket with one hand with the ball inside.

· Rattle the ball loosely inside your hand, as if you were shaking dice. (See figure 1.3.)

· Switch hands, rattle those dice

· Drop the ball from one hand to the other, back and forth.

· Catch the ball in a loose hand, not tight.

· Just three or four inches apart will do, more if you like.

· Now keep dropping back and forth *but with your eyes closed.*

· Notice that each hand "knows" where the other hand is without using your eyes.

· Open your eyes.

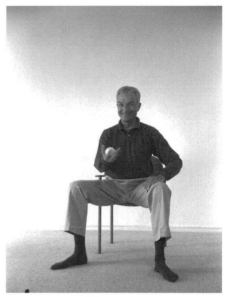

Figure 1.3

EXERCISE 1.4
The Candle

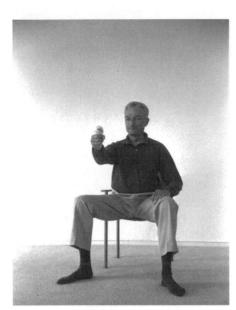

Figure 1.4

- Make a fist like you are holding a candle.
- Place the ball on top of the fist like it was the candle. (See figure 1.4.)
- Move the ball/candle all around: hold the candle as if you are looking high and low and around to each side in a dark room.
- Now move it around with your eyes closed.
- Change hands and repeat these steps.
- Now holding the ball/candle on top of your fist.
- Open your fist slowly and let the ball slip down into your palm.
- Now squeeze the ball back up to the candle position.
- Do this with your eyes closed.
- Notice that your hand knows how to balance the ball without your eyes helping.

EXERCISE 1.5
The Ladybug

· Put one hand out flat, palm down.

· Use your other hand to place the ball on the back of your fingers.

· If you press down your middle finger slightly, you can make a little cradle for the ball.

· Balance the ball on the back of your hand like a pet ladybug. (See figure 1.5.)

· Move your arm and hand all around, show everybody your pet ladybug.

· Now toss the ball up, turn your hand over, and catch it.

· Change hands, do it again.

· Then back and forth: left hand, ladybug, catch; right hand, ladybug, catch; and so on.

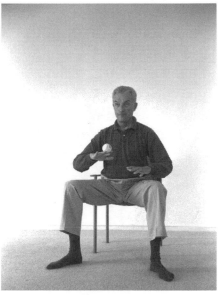

Figure 1.5

EXERCISE 1.6
Hand Dance

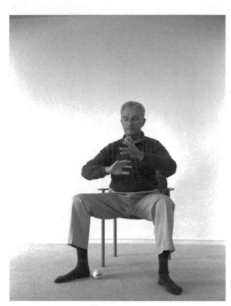

Figure 1.6

- Now put the ball on the floor.
- Put your hand out flat, palm down.
- Balance an *imaginary* ball on the back of your hand.
- Feel your hand from the inside holding the imaginary ball.
- Close your eyes.
- Keep feeling your hand from the inside.
- Notice you can feel it more clearly with your eyes closed.
- Roll your hand over and let the imaginary ball drop to the floor.
- With your eyes closed, move your hand one finger at a time.
- Eyes still closed, turn your hand over and back.
- Pay attention to the inside of your hand, your wrist, your arm.
- Notice each joint, each bone, each muscle, each tiny difference inside your hand. Feel your skin from the inside stretching and relaxing.
- Eyes closed, pay attention as your hand opens, closes, turns, spreads, reaches, pulls back, or just moves slowly and gracefully in the air, like a jellyfish in the water, or like smoke drifting up from a campfire. (See figure 1.6.)
- This is "Hand Dancing." Enjoy it. Let it be beautiful to you.
- After five minutes, open your eyes slowly and look around you.
- Have you been "away" for a little while?

When you look at your hand from the inside you become aware what a miracle the hand is. How delicate and sensitive, how cleverly constructed, what a marvelous living machine! And what an infinite number of moves the hand can make, what an infinite number of sensations come to you from inside your hand: now moving, now still, now tight, now loose, now warm, now cool, now strong, now weak, moving up here, but down there, and on and on. Dancing your hands with your eyes closed, there are so many variations that you soon run out of words! All a person can do is just marvel at the flood of information coming into your mind from your miraculous hand.

Kinesthesia

This concept is very important. That inward sensation of your hand that you can feel more clearly when your eyes are closed and your mind is quiet is called *kinesthesia*. Here's how the *American Heritage Dictionary* defines it:

> The sensation of bodily position, presence, or movement resulting chiefly from stimulation of sensory nerve endings in muscles, tendons, and joints.

Kinesthesia is every bit as much a "sense" as the five senses we usually think of: sight, hearing, smell, taste, and touch. Just as each sense has a sense organ—eyes for sight, ears for hearing, skin for touch—kinesthesia is sensed through receptors that are designed to pick up specific kinds of information: there are kinesthetic receptors inside muscle tissue that report how tight or loose the muscle is contracted; there are special nerve endings lining the sockets at each joint that tell how bent or straight the joint is; and there are nerve points along the tracks where tendons run that register tension and warn of danger—like when we get that unfunny whack on our funnybone. All these kinesthetic organs pick up stimulation and send messages along nerve pathways to our brains. Therefore, we must recognize that kinesthesia is a sense.

It is a unique sense, however. The familiar five senses report on what's happening *outside* our bodies, more or less, while kinesthesia reports on something happening *inside* our bodies. When you close your eyes and turn your hand palm up and then palm down you can tell the difference. You can tell the difference even though you are not looking at your hand nor touching anything around you. How do you *know* your hand is palm up? And now palm down? That sense inside your arm and hand—the sense that knows where your hand is and whether it is up or down, open or closed—that is your kinesthesia.

Keep your attention focused on your kinesthesia during workouts. When you begin the exercise routine, bring your attention to what you are doing and then to the interior feeling of what you are doing.

Now, if you are like me, your mind will wander off pretty quickly. It's like the old joke: "I am of two minds, but one of them is lost, and the other one is out looking for it." When you notice your mind wandering, gently return your attention to what you are doing and then to the interior feeling of what you are doing. Kinesthesia is like the bull's-eye on a target, while everything else you might think of is like the rings around the bull's-eye. When you notice your attention has wandered off the bull's-eye to one of the rings, gently correct your aim back to the bull's-eye. Kinesthesia, the sense of your body from the inside, is where your attention belongs during your workout. This is home base.

Spine and Breathing Warm-up

The next set of exercises will focus on loosening your spine and, at the same time, deepening your breathing. The two are related: a stiff spine prevents you from breathing fully, and breathing shallowly lets your spine get stiff. The ancient art of hatha yoga teaches spinal undulation coupled with full tidal breathing in one of its most basic exercises, *The Salute to the Sun* (it's meant to be done first thing in the morning at the rising of the sun). The exercises below derive from the *Salute*, but are adapted to the needs of people with Parkinson's.

Full Tidal Breathing

Breath can be said to have a "tide"; like the ocean tide, it comes in, it goes out—sometimes just a little, sometimes a lot. You want "a lot"! Every time you breathe a full inhale and then a full exhale your whole spine *undulates* from top to tail. The spine is *designed* to undulate, your spine loves to undulate, everything works better when your spine undulates. That undulation works like a pump to move all the essential fluids inside your body in a helpful direction: fresh blood out from the heart, used blood back toward the heart and lungs.

We must have learned to breathe at the shoreline. We have all been breathing and undulating like the sea since our ancestors crawled out of the waves and up onto the shore. If you close your eyes and imagine lying on the shore of some ancient sea—your head toward the land, your legs still lying in the waves—you may be able to feel your breath as a tide. The tide flows in from below up toward your heart and head, then drains back out to sea as your exhale. That's your **full tidal breathing** and these next exercises will encourage you to notice how it moves.

You may think it odd that some of your breathing exercises start with a full *exhale* instead of a full *inhale*. Notice that your exercise actually starts when you "sit forward at the edge of your chair." When you sit upright and at rest, your lungs are more full of breath than they are empty! *Taking in* a big breath is just topping off an already full tank. Therefore, your first effort, whether it is a push or a bend, will help to push as much air *out* of your lungs as possible. Then when you come back up to sitting upright, your lungs will fill again "by themselves." **For full tidal breathing, the effort part of the breath cycle is *the exhale*; the relaxation part of the breath cycle is *the inhale.*** This may feel unfamiliar at first, but take it from a man who has taught acting for thirty five years. When you want to shift into full tidal breathing, make an effort on the exhale to push all your breath out, then relax and *allow* your breath to come in by itself on the inhale. Effort on exhale; relax on inhale.

EXERCISE 1.7
Spine Forward and Back

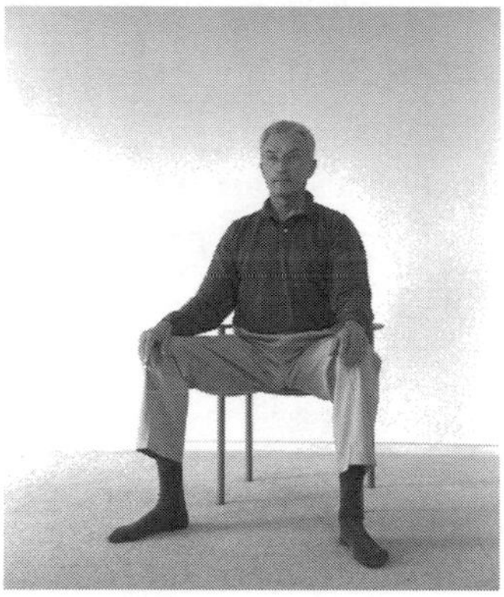

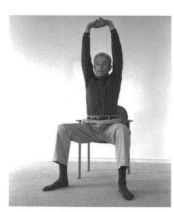

Figure 1.7a

- Sit forward on the front edge of your chair.
- Place your feet as wide apart as possible. (See figure 1.7a.)
- Lace your fingers in a prayer position.
- Stick your thumbs up.
- Now rotate wrists inward to stick your thumbs down.
- Push your hands forward till your elbows come straight. (See figure 1.7b.)

- Breathe out a full breath as you push.
- Lift your arms high overhead, keeping your palms pressed away from you. (See figure 1.7c.)
- Breathe in through your nostrils the biggest breath possible.

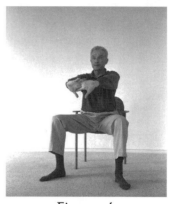

Figure 1.7b

Figure 1.7c

- Feel your ribs expand and your upper back arch upward.
- Bring your arms forward and down.
- Separate your hands when they reach waist level.
- Now reach down to the floor between your feet. (See figure 1.7d.)
- Keep your elbows inside your knees.

· Press outward against your legs with the back of your arms.

· Breathe out through pursed lips all the breath you have and more.

· Reach down as far as you can, then go another quarter inch.

· Drop your head and look back under your chair "to see if anyone stuck any chewing gum under the front edge."

· Come to rest for a moment.

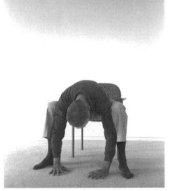

Figure 1.7d

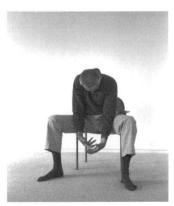

Figure 1.7e

· Pick up an imaginary baby. (See figure 1.7e.)

· Bring her up, kiss her head, and put her in your heart.

· Breathe in as you come up; let your breath come in through your nostrils.

· Sit balanced and upright in your chair.

· Come to rest for a moment, hands on your thighs, palms upward. Breathe out completely.

· Lace your fingers and begin the upward stretch again.

· Repeat the upward and downward stretch five times.

Notice that you can go a little farther up and a little farther down each time. That means your muscles and spine are lengthening and opening little by little as you keep asking them firmly and gently to lengthen, open, reach, and then relax. Let's say you are able to go just another quarter of an inch toward the floor each time you bend forward: after five repetitions you will have gained a full inch and a quarter!

A word about "picking up the baby." First, of course, imaginary baby boys work just as well for the purpose as imaginary baby girls. (If you can't stand babies, any imaginary small treasure will do just as well: a keepsake, a kitten, a dividend check.) The purpose is to invite you to cradle and protect the imaginary bundle in that special way people do. Most likely you will shift your feet to be sure of your footing; you will reach your arms all the way down to the floor; your hands will stay close together in front of you as they form a tiny cradle; you will bend your lower back, tuck your backside under, and bring the baby "inside" the curved safety of your whole body; you will keep your head down as you gaze at the baby while lifting her. Only after you have put the baby safely "into your heart" will you let your attention shift out to the world around you.

You've just learned the CORRECT way to come up! By protecting the baby you are protecting yourself from back strain, neck strain, dizziness, and distraction!

You can prove this to yourself by trying the opposite of each of the above. Bend down inside your knees again. Then before you start up, raise your head, straighten your back, put your arms out to each side, look all around to see if anybody is watching, and sit right up. You will probably notice the strain in your lower back. There may also be a strain in your shoulders and neck. If you come up fast enough, you may notice a bit of dizziness as the blood pressure in your head drops for a moment. Most likely your breath will be held as you rise and will come exploding out of you once you are all the way up.

Taken all together, these incorrect ways to come up can make the movement seem difficult, if not painful. And when you do this five times in a row, the difficulty will only get worse.

We will revisit "picking up the baby" in many other exercises throughout this book. It will become one of the most useful of all your movement strategies.

Herbert Jacobsen built highways and bridges and hydroelectric dams most of his life. He was usually the supervising engineer, but no one would doubt for a minute he could do any hard physical job he asked another man to do. He is still a big man, broad across the shoulders, with huge hands and a slow and generous smile.

And he loves to eat; no one would doubt that, either. His Parkinson's does not cause tremor very often. Nor is his balance much affected. He moves with that curious grace some very large men seem blessed with, but he moves *slowly*. Parkinson's has made him stiff almost everywhere. He is usually sore in his shoulders and neck and in his calves.

Stretching is not Herb's favorite exercise, but it is the one he needs the most. So he does these stretches, slowly and deliberately. When I tell him it is okay to complain out loud while he does them, he looks at me ruefully and chuckles. So he groans a bit and grunts now and then, and he keeps going. When I tell him he should keep stretching and someday he will be able to touch the floor, he says, in his Old Country accent, "Ya, someday," meaning never. It took him fourteen months, but now he can touch the floor. Big tendons take more time to stretch.

EXERCISE 1.8
Spine Rotation

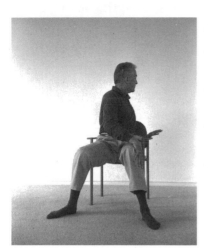

Figure 1.8a

- Sit forward on the front edge of your chair.
- Sitting upright, twist around to your LEFT and look directly behind you. (See figure 1.8a.)
- Use your hands to grasp the arm and the back of the chair to help pull yourself around.
- Breathe out through pursed lips all the breath you have and a little more.
- You will feel this stretch strongest in your waist and neck, a little less in your upper back.
- Turn back around to center, breathing in deeply through your nose.

- Come to rest for a moment.
- Now twist to your RIGHT and look directly behind you. (See figure 1.8b.)
- Breathe out through pursed lips all the breath you have and a little more.
- Turn back around to center, taking in a full breath.
- Come to rest for a moment.
- Repeat both the LEFT twist and the RIGHT twist five times.

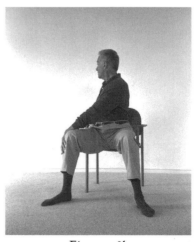

Figure 1.8b

EXERCISE 1.9
Spine Rotation and Bending

- Sit forward on the front edge of your chair.
- Reach your LEFT hand down to the LEFT side of your chair, with a full out-breath. (See figure 1.9a.)
- Look right next to the back leg of your chair.
- Catch an imaginary mouse.
- Rise back up to center, with a full in-breath.
- Come to rest for a moment.
- Reach your RIGHT hand down to the RIGHT side of your chair, with a full out-breath. (See figure 1.9b.)

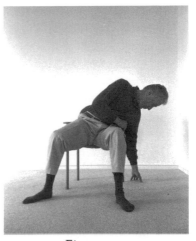

Figure 1.9a

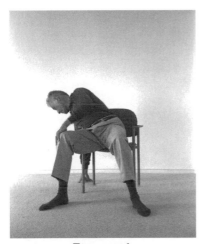

Figure 1.9b

- Look right next to the back leg of your chair.
- Catch the mouse's wife, next to the back leg of your chair.
- Be sure your neck and head are bent, "looking for the mouse."
- Enjoy that stretch in your neck and shoulders.
- Rise back up to center, with a full in-breath.
- Come to rest for a moment.
- Repeat LEFT and RIGHT, at least five times.
- Each time, let the weight of your head stretch your neck.
- Come to rest.

You may find yourself glad for a moment's rest. Now you are ready to finish your warm-up. The grand finale will consist of a free-form, eyes-closed, noisy stretch in every direction. People stretch wholeheartedly like this at the beginning of the day when they first get up after a good night's sleep. People also stretch and groan like this at the end of a day's work. You may need to fake it for a little while, but usually after a few fake noises, you will find yourself connecting with some really satisfying groans and grunts.

This free and noisy stretch is called *Groaner's Yoga* to make clear that it should be totally playful and irreverent to the highest degree. (Yoga classes are usually conducted in total, reverent silence, except for the teacher's instructions.) Make the atmosphere of your workouts irreverent, noisy, sloppy, comic, and totally free.

Easy Does It; But Do It

Exercises will be more enjoyable if you allow yourself to do them within a mood of general playfulness, relaxation, and irreverence. Grunt, groan, complain, tell jokes, and tease yourself and your exercise friends. Don't get too precise and serious about doing everything just right. Clown it up a little. This easy playfulness releases some of the rigidity in your muscles, and the irreverent attitude banishes some of the mental and emotional stress that can make your PD symptoms worse.

Your motto ought to be: "Easy does it; but do it." Combining relaxation with exercise is a basic principle throughout this book. It derives from Tai Chi Chuan and hatha yoga, in which conditioning the body takes place in a calm and serene atmosphere. The exercises in this book are *not* calisthenics; they are *not* rock-and-roll aerobics; they are *not* boot camp with Sergeant Toughguy. You want to combine effort with relaxation. Easy does it; but do it.

EXERCISE 1.10
Groaner's Yoga

· Sit forward and at ease.

· Close your eyes.

· Join your hands and lift them high overhead.

· Stretch and groan.

· Keep your eyes closed.

· Turn you hands loose and stretch and twist and reach and groan in every direction. Let it all hang out. (It helps if everybody in the room gets into the same noisy stretching.)

When you do an ordinary, getting-out-of-bed-in-the-morning stretch with your arms out and up, you may even find it quite natural to yawn. If a yawn comes, let it come and get into it; then yawn and yawn till your tears flow and make lots of yawning sounds. That is all to the good, because your next lesson begins with just that: the ordinary, garden-variety yawn!

Summary

Your workout hour begins with a few easy sitting exercises:

• First you work with a tennis ball to sensitize and wake up your feet.

• Then you take the tennis ball into your hands and use it to stretch your hands and practice some small motor skills.

• Three spine stretches come next: a long stretch forward and back, then a twist stretch to rotate your spine, and finally a twist and drop stretch to loosen your upper back and neck.

- You finish with *Groaner's Yoga*: stretch and groan over and over till you get into really satisfying groans.

Every bit as important for your overall success with this exercise program is your grasp of the four key ideas presented in this first lesson:

- As you work out, you should push each exercise to your personal **hurts good** point, and no further.

- Your attention should remain centered on your **kinesthesia**, the shifting pattern of sensations coming to you from inside your body.

- You want to adjust your breathing during the workout session to **full tidal breathing**, allowing for a long exhale of each breath followed by a complete inhale.

- Finally, try to develop a general mood of playfulness, ease, and relaxation as you work out. Within that relaxed mood, you should focus your effort on each exercise. **Easy does it; but do it.**

As you go forward in this book and learn the rest of the workout, you will find many reminders of these principles. You may want to write them out with a big marker and post them where you can see them. To be brief:

Hurts good

Kinesthesia

Full breathing

Easy does it; but do it

Lesson 2

Voice and Speech (The Cooldown)

About half of all the people with Parkinson's disease will develop some problem with voice and speech: they may speak too softly to be heard, they may speak in a monotone, they may develop a hoarse voice. Words may be crowded together so their meaning is lost; the endings of words—their final consonant sounds—may be dropped; sentences may be broken into short, staccato fragments. People with PD may find it difficult to initiate speech and find themselves pausing just as they are about to reply to a question or make a comment; and a listener may respond to that pause by thinking the speaker is befuddled. There are even some times when the ability to speak may completely disappear for a while.

Communication suffers under all these limitations. Many people say that this loss of communication is the most painful of all their PD difficulties. They become frustrated when asked to repeat themselves over and over again. They fear talking with strangers. Sometimes they withdraw from social settings altogether, because they feel that they cannot make a contribution or that they slow down the conversation. The resultant social isolation, loneliness, and the feelings of uselessness can become quite painful.

Richard Ellis takes an active role in a group at his church called the Elders. He likes to help people with their problems, and he devotes himself to acquiring wisdom, a task he feels is appropriate for a man well into his eighties. He has a knack for making people around him feel they are somehow special. People want to hear what he has to say and often seek him out to settle conflicts or to help them make choices. He has written several books during his long life and usually has something interesting to say. But that's where the trouble starts.

Parkinson's disease causes Richard's speech to be very difficult to understand. His problem seems to vary from day to day, so he can never be sure when his speech will work and when it will not. On a bad day, his wife needs to ask him to repeat himself after every sentence.

Richard's words trip over themselves. He may start out to say, "I met a fellow who has a new boat over in Sausalito," but what comes out is more like, "Meafela whosa bone oven salto." He can slow himself way down and say one word at a time, and it improves to, "Ah, met, a fella, over, insausalito, who has, a new, boat." If a listener looks directly into Richard's face, the meaning comes across.

To counteract voice and speech difficulties, you need to learn to speak like an actor. You need to speak slowly, clearly, and distinctly. Slowing down your speech will actually speed up your communication: *you will not lose time by having to repeat yourself.* Your breathing needs to be deep and strong. You need a long, strong out-breath to power your words and finish your sentences all the way to the end. You need to make your lips, teeth, tongue, and jaw move with exaggerated precision to shape and project every sound in every part of every word. And you need to encourage your face to express meanings and feelings that can be seen clear across the room, or as actors say, "clear to the last row."

Your overall goal is *communication.* You need to do whatever it takes to get your meaning across. The show must go on. You want to be understood. You also need to listen well; you want the other person to know that you understand what has been said to you. You do not want to withdraw to the sidelines. So speak gracefully, mindfully, and completely. Speak like an actor.

All the exercises below derive from basic actor training. The ones suggested here are traditional parts of almost every voice-training system. Beginning actors learn them the first week of voice class. Most actors will run through some variation of these exercises before every rehearsal and performance. And actors will continue to practice every day, even when they are not working, to keep their "instrument" in condition. As a person with Parkinson's, you will need to do the same.

Exercises for Stronger Voice Production

You begin your voice work with a short session of the exercise you did at the end of Lesson 1, *Groaner's Yoga*. With your whole body, take a few minutes of free stretching, twisting, and reaching. Go past your usual limits to the place where your muscles "hurt good" and your joints get a good pull. Through all of this, let your voice grunt and groan with the effort. A certain amount of playacting is expected with this. After a bit of faking, you'll find the groove, and more realistic groans will come naturally.

Those natural grunts and groans that escape you when you really get into a good stretching session can be called part of your *natural voice*. Your natural voice comes from a more primitive, more physical part of you than does your normal, everyday voice. What you feel in your muscles comes directly out through your voice without editing or affectation, and often without any interference from your Parkinson's. You don't really have to ask yourself to describe what's happening in words; the noise you make *is* the description of what's happening. You will find a strong connection with that natural voice in several of the exercises in this lesson. The first will be a very familiar sound: the big, open-throated "AHHH" sound of a Yawn.

The Theory and Practice of the Yawn

Some neurologists will tell you that you cannot yawn on command. In their understanding, a yawn is an involuntary reaction controlled by the *autonomic nervous system*. The autonomic nervous system regulates involuntary functions in two major ways: it accelerates your body for "fight or flight" (sympathetic mode) or it slows your body for "rest and relaxation" (parasympathetic mode). Activities controlled by this system include sweating, shivering, hiccuping, the flow of tears from your eyes, the speeding up and slowing down of your heartbeat, the opening or narrowing of blood vessels, and even the dilation of your pupils. All of these functions are very important for fighting-and-fleeing and resting-and-relaxing, and all are outside our conscious control; hence autonomic (from the Greek *autonomos*, meaning "self-ruling").

The neurologists are correct as far as they go. But though a real yawn may not be *commanded*, it can be *invited*. By going through the following steps, most people can bring on a real yawn. Try this right now as you read through these suggestions:

- Suggest to yourself that it sure would be nice to have a big old yawn right about now.

- Give yourself permission to take in a large inhale through your wide open mouth. Just open your mouth and start breathing in right now.

- Pull your arms back and to the sides and then lift them up over your head and roll your shoulders to loosen them.

- You may start to yawn and not quite make it.

- Make a big *pretend* yawn sound.

- Pretend to yawn several times with bigger and bigger *pretend* yawn sounds.

- Cover your mouth out of pretend politeness.

- And then, oh bliss, here comes a real yawn!

- Feel it coming. Feel that *involuntary* lift in your ribcage and that *involuntary* stretching in your throat, your eyes perhaps squeeze shut ... and, finally, you go over the top.

- A REAL YAWN! Very satisfying.

So there you have it. You fake yawn till you make it real. For a little while *you* do the yawn, and then *the yawn* does you! You pretend to do the action—and then the real action comes. (You have just learned one of the great secrets of the art of acting! Actors pretend they mean it for a while, then somehow they find they really do mean it.)

Yawning is contagious. If you are with other people when you yawn, especially if you just happen to yawn a little bit out loud, then the fun begins. Pretty soon, other people in the group will start to yawn, too! Soon the whole bunch of you are yawning like sea lions on a sunny beach. Depending on the circumstances, this can be quite hilarious.

By pretending to yawn you have invited the real yawn. By giving yourself permission to yawn in a group, you have invited everyone else in the group to likewise give themselves permission to yawn. The neurologists may be right that you cannot *command* a yawn; but your own experience proves that a real yawn can be *invited.*

EXERCISE 2.1
The Vocalized Yawn

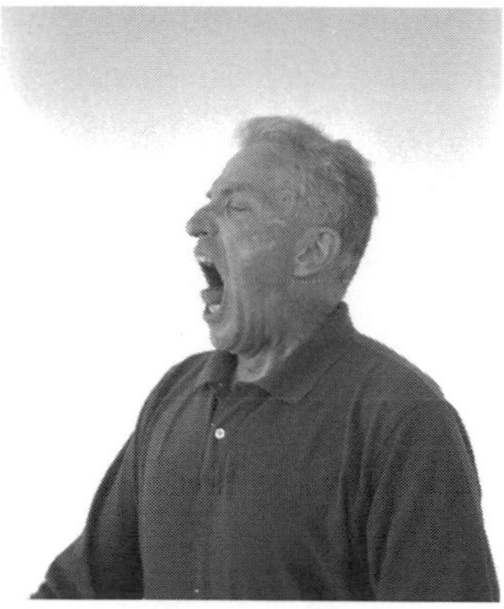

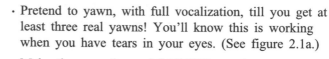

- Pretend to yawn, with full vocalization, till you get at least three real yawns! You'll know this is working when you have tears in your eyes. (See figure 2.1a.)

- Make the open-throated "AHHH" sound.

- Spread open your hands in the "catcher's mitt" stretch you learned in the tennis ball exercises.

- Notice that the stretching of your hands feels similar to the stretching of your throat that happens in the midst of a real yawn.

- Feel your hand and throat widening at the same time.

Figure 2.1a

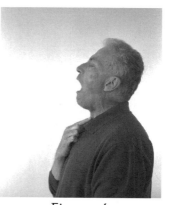

Figure 2.1b

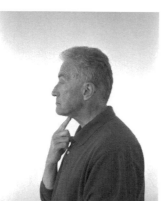

- Feel your larynx with your fingers. Notice that your larynx is in its lowest possible position during a yawn. (See figure 2.1b.)

- Then feel your larynx move up to its highest position with a swallow. (See figure 2.1c.)

- Larynx down with a yawn; larynx up with a swallow.

Figure 2.1c

PD causes many difficulties connected with the throat: diminished breathing, soft speech, monotone speech, hoarseness, high-pitched squeaky voice, and, last but not least, difficulty with swallowing. *The Vocalized Yawn* is one of the simplest, easiest, most effective exercises to reduce all of these difficulties. That is why you need to integrate it into all the exercise routines presented in this book. You will find explicit instructions to "do a yawn" at many points throughout this book. But don't limit yourself to the explicit; yawn ad lib, as we say in the theater. While exercising, yawn at your liberty, yawn whenever you like, but yawn *often*. The mighty Yawn! Don't leave home without it.

You are hereby initiated into the Society of Professional Yawners. Your membership entitles you to yawn morning, noon, and night, in the presence of politicians, preachers, pundits, and all other kinds of important people; except your spouse, of course, spouses require special negotiations. Probably the best way is to invite them to join the Society. You may confer full membership, with all rights and privileges, on anyone whom you can persuade to share a hearty yawn with you. Yawning feels good. Because you have Parkinson's disease, you need to become an inveterate yawner, a compulsive yawner, an over-the-top, outrageous, expert yawner! You need to do it because you have Parkinson's; so enjoy it.

The Benefits of Yawning

There are four important reasons why yawning needs to be practiced so thoroughly.

- Yawning promotes the deepest possible diaphragmatic *breathing*.

- Yawning trains you to open your throat so you can speak *with full volume*.

- Yawning exercises your throat muscles in a way that improves *swallowing*.

- Yawning allows you to *relax* your muscles while working out.

Let's discuss each of these benefits in turn. Yawning is very important, so you need to thoroughly convince yourself that frequent yawning is an essential health practice.

Breathing

People with PD have a special difficulty because the muscles of the throat and chest usually have the same PD symptoms that the legs and hands have: rigidity, slowness of movement, and incomplete range of execution. As a result, most people with PD breathe shallowly. Yawning opens all the airways and stretches all the muscles that you need for deep breathing.

The ability to breathe deeply and fully can also help a person whose dyskinesia seems to cause rapid jerks in breath rhythm. Breathing with long, yawning inhales followed by vocalizing with long, complete exhales can help to calm and organize such disordered movements into a centered easiness.

It would be an exaggeration to say that shallow breathing causes depression. It would also be an exaggeration to say that deep breathing cures depression. Still, you may have noticed that a bit of aerobic exercise can dispel a stubborn gloom, or that a rousing hymn can bring enthusiasm to a droopy congregation. The deep breathing involved in such practices clearly changes people's moods for the better. You will have a chance to check this out in the next exercise, *Singing on AHHHH.*

Speaking

Parkinson's causes a loss of voice power and a variety of speech difficulties in many people with the disease. Voice volume is lost because the chest and diaphragm do not expand fully when a person takes in a breath. The chest and diaphragm act as a bellows that forces air through the vocal cords to produce sound. They need to have an ample supply of air to do their job.

Pitch problems—monotony, hoarseness, and squeakiness—center inside the larynx at the vocal cords. Sound is produced by the rapid opening and closing of the vocal cords as air is forced through them. The cords may open wide but not close well; then you have a whispery voice. The cords may not open well or close too strongly; then you get hoarseness. Monotony—the absence of pitch variation—comes from rigidity in the whole larynx area. A yawn fills the lungs, stretches the muscles around the larynx, and opens the vocal cords, and the open-throated AHHHH sound exercises the natural voice through a wide range of pitches and volumes.

Swallowing

Many people with PD will experience difficulties with swallowing. You may have difficulty getting pills down. You may sometimes inhale food and liquids into your larynx (aspiration), which will cause you to choke and cough and alarm the people you're with.

Yawning contracts the muscles that move the larynx into its most downward position. The only way they can do this is to stretch the muscles that raise the larynx to its most upward position when you swallow. At the same time, the yawn stretches wide the muscles of the throat, the very ones that have to contract strongly when you swallow. The Yawn can be thought of as the reciprocal movement to the Swallow: the better the yawn, the better the swallow.

Yawning promotes flexibility in all the muscles you need for efficient swallowing. People who practice yawning every day often discover that they stop drooling.

Relaxation

PD tightens your muscles. Yawning is an important part of your workout because it helps you relax your muscles at the same time you are stretching them. Relaxation of your entire body is governed by the autonomic nervous system. Now here's the trick: yawning *shifts* the autonomic nervous system from the sympathetic "fight or flight" mode to the parasympathetic "rest and relaxation" mode.

During your workout, you need to maintain a general mood of ease and relaxation; each exercise calls on you to focus your effort and attention on a specific action *within* that general mood of relaxation. Yawning all through your workout will encourage you to maintain the proper combination of calm serenity and wholehearted effort that leads to gracefulness.

In conclusion: Yawn noisily, wholeheartedly, and often! End of sermon.

The next exercise will be as easy as pie. You are going to sing three verses of any three songs you know the tune of, but you don't have to remember any of the words. How's that for easy? No words at all! No words allowed! You sing all three verses of all three songs using only that wonderful open-throated AHHHH you learned to do with your yawning.

EXERCISE 2.2
Singing On AHHH

· Sit forward on the edge of your chair, knees wide, head high.

· Open your throat as if you are going to yawn, but don't yawn.

· Just make the yawn sound, the open throated AHHHH.

· Hold AHHHH on a singing pitch for a moment or two.

· Pretend to be a great opera singer tuning up!

· Then choose a song, and sing three verses on AHHHH.

· Ahhh Ah Ah Ah Ah Ah Ahhh Ah . . . (This is supposed to be the first line of "I've Been Working on the Railroad." Yeah, pretty feeble, but you get the idea.)

· Keep it open, keep it loud, and keep it going.

· Choose another song, sing three verses on AHHHH.

· Choose a third song, sing three verses on AHHHH.

Make this plenty of fun. Be a great comic opera star. You may be surprised at how hard it is to keep going, but keep going just the same. Keep your throat open to make your AHHHH as much like a vocalized yawn as possible. If you find yourself actually yawning in the middle of a song, *you are doing it just right!*

Here's a short list of songs to get you started:

"I've Been Working on the Railroad"
"London Bridge Is Falling Down"
"Old Macdonald Had a Farm"
"Jingle Bells"
"Deck the Halls"
"Joy to the World"
"Down in the Valley"
"Oh Suzanna!"
"Amazing Grace"

"A Mighty Fortress Is Our God"
"We Shall Overcome"
"Man on the Flying Trapeze"
"When the Saints Go Marching In"
"Night and Day"
"Chattanooga Choo Choo"
"Oh What a Beautiful Morning"
"Some Enchanted Evening"
"Don't Fence Me In"
"No Business Like Show Business"

As soon as you finish singing the third song, try speaking in a normal tone. You may be surprised at the increased volume of your voice. You may find that your ability to complete a whole sentence in one breath has suddenly returned. That's the simple point of this exercise: to improve the power of your voice by increasing the amount of breath power available at each breath. If you don't feel improvement right away, don't worry. After a few weeks practice you'll be impressed with the results. But practice daily!

You may be a bit tired after three songs. Notice *where* you feel the tiredness. You may feel a little sore in your rib cage, or just under your rib cage at your diaphragm. The effort of singing has exercised the bellows of your ribs and diaphragm to increase the volume of air with each breath.

Exercises for Increased Facial Mobility and Articulation

A good voice comes from an **open throat** and **full breathing**. Two other factors are involved in improved communication: **lively facial expressions** and **clear articulation** of your words. These clown faces will stretch your face every which way. You will also find more of your natural voice in the emotional sounds of crying, laughter, growling, and screaming.

EXERCISE 2.3
Four Clown Faces

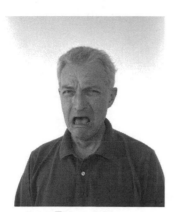

Figure 2.3a

- Make your face into each of the following clown faces.
- Make sure you really grimace and exaggerate.
- Find sounds that fit the emotion of the facial expression.
- Carry that sound as far as you can go. Keep going with each face for a full minute.

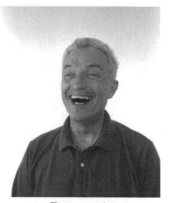

Figure 2.3b

- The Sad Clown: *Grief*—Mouth turned down, sad eyes, whimper, sob, wail. (See figure 2.3a.)
- The Happy Clown: *Joy*—Big smile, beaming eyes, giggles, laugh. (See figure 2.3b.)
- The Angry Clown: *Anger*—Scowl, glare, show your teeth, growl, roar. (See figure 2.3c.)

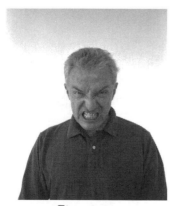

Figure 2.3c

- The Timid Clown: *Fear*—Mouth wide, eyes wide, eyebrows high, get ready to scream, strangled scream, open scream (so long as you don't frighten the neighbors!). (See figure 2.3d.)

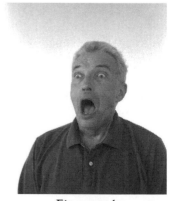

Figure 2.3d

Articulators

These next exercises will stretch and stimulate your **lips**, **teeth**, **tongue**, and **jaw**. You will focus your attention into these parts of your mouth as you go. You need to wake up these articulators and then ask them to exaggerate their shaping of vowels and consonants.

Some of these drills may seem pretty silly, but they do work in promoting your sensory awareness in the mouth area. That's what you need, you need to *feel* all the parts of your mouth making words come out clearly. These should do the job.

Exercise 2.4
Lips, Teeth, Tongue, and Jaw

Pronounce these words carefully several times: "Lips, Teeth, Tongue, and Jaw." Notice how the names of each one actually uses the part named.

· Feel "lips" touch when you speak their name.

· Watch how your tongue touches your teeth when you say "teeth."

· Your tongue moves when you say "tongue."

· And your jaw drops open when you say "jaw."

· Now concentrate on making sounds with each part of your mouth.

· Have fun with these sounds.

Lips:

· Flubber your lips like a motorcycle revving its engine.

· Try a "razzberry," with your tongue between your lips; this is also known as a Bronx cheer.

· Do Fish Lips, protruding your lips like a goldfish feeding.

· Make kissing sounds—smack smack smack.

Teeth:

· Feel your tongue touch your teeth when you say "this, that, with, earth." Exaggerate the tongue touch with the "th" sounds.

· Feel your lip touch your teeth as you say "father finds fresh fish off soft reef." Exaggerate the lip touch with the "fa" sounds. Feel your breath hiss through your teeth on the "sh" sounds.

Tongue:

· Push your tongue as far out of your mouth as possible.

· Trill your tongue.

· Curl your tongue as you would for a spitball.

· Feel your tongue move forward and pull back as you say "EE YA EE YA EE YA!" Exaggerate the forward-and-back movement.

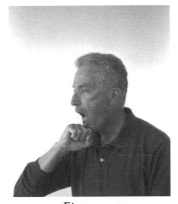

Figure 2.4

Jaw:

· Massage your jaw muscles using the knuckles of your fist.

· Drop your jaw with a "Duhh" sound and a stupid expression.

· Rap your chin downward with the edge of your fist till you feel your jaw loosen. (See figure 2.4.)

Now that your articulators are warmed up, you'll put it all together.

EXERCISE 2.5
Over-Articulation

Read out this familiar chant from *Jack and the Beanstalk:*

Fee, Fie, Fo, Fum!
I smell the blood of an Englishman.
Be he alive or be he dead
I'll grind his bones to make my bread.

· Use your lips, teeth, tongue, and jaw in a completely exaggerated way.

· Move your lips a lot.

· Make the lips-to-teeth and tongue-to-teeth touches very strong and noisy.

· Make your vowel sounds long; draw them out.

· Open your mouth very wide as you say the words, so wide that two of your knuckles will fit inside your front teeth.

The following exercise will help you practice communicating: speaking *and* listening. This can help you build up your confidence as you work to speak gracefully, mindfully, and completely.

EXERCISE 2.6
The Echo Exercise

Select a piece of writing. It can be a children's book, a poem, a story, a soliloquy from Shakespeare, the Gettysburg Address, the First Amendment, the Song of Songs, the Twenty-third Psalm, or any other work you are familiar with. It really helps a lot if you truly enjoy the material.

· Read or recite your piece to another person.

· Read one line of poetry at a time.

· With prose, break long sentences into meaningful phrases.

· Speak one line or phrase so clearly that your partner can repeat back what you say, word for word.

· Listen carefully as they say it back to you.

· If they make even the slightest mistake, that means you have not pronounced that word clearly enough.

· Go back and say the line again, *over-articulating* the word (or words) they had trouble with.

· When they get it right, go on with your reading. Speak the next line or phrase very clearly. Listen as your partner says it back. And so on.

You may want to read using your finger on the page to keep track of your place. That moving finger can also help you keep your reading pace *slow* enough to say each word completely—the beginning, the middle, and the end (including that darned final consonant)—before you start the next word.

You will not only need to *speak* clearly to make this work. You will also need to *listen* carefully to the other person repeat your words back to you. You need to look at the person as you speak and keep watching them as they say the words back to you. Only when you know they have it right may you go on. By listening carefully to the other person, you model for them how you want them to listen to you. The quality of your listening sets the standard for your conversation. What goes around comes around. One of the highest compliments one actor can give another is, "You listen well."

Here's a tip: stick with the same poem or story or prayer through many, many repetitions. Actors work on short pieces like these—they use them as audition pieces—sometimes for years. As you work on your piece week after week, you will notice how the meaning of each word and the feelings within each word become clearer to you as you try to make them clearer to your listener. Try different listeners. Try tape-recording your piece, so you can become your own listener. In time, the meanings, feelings, and images that are waiting there in the words will find their way out through your voice. You will "become one with the words." Hard to describe this, but, like love, you'll know it when it happens. It's very satisfying.

Summary

Your voice and speech workout started with several **vocalized yawns**, to open your throat and lungs and free up your natural voice. Then you took the open-throated AHHHH from your yawning practice and sang three songs without the words.

- Singing on AHHHH exercises your diaphragm, chest, and throat to promote **full tidal breathing**—a deep strong exhale and a full easy inhale.

- That full tidal breathing gives you the powerful air capacity you need to speak full sentences, and to speak them loud enough for folks to hear you.

Your **articulation** work started with *Four Clown Faces* to stretch and enliven your face muscles:

- Your emotional play with your face reminds you to allow yourself to express feelings when you communicate.

- You will learn to counteract the wooden face of PD with a bit of conscious acting to let people see your inner liveliness.

Next you did sensitization exercises for your lips, teeth, tongue, and jaw so that you could exaggerate the articulation of every vowel and every consonant as you spoke:

- You need to feel your lips, teeth, tongue, and jaw go through those articulation movements so that your words will be clear and complete, rather than jumbled or truncated.

Finally you learned an echo exercise.

- You read your selected piece to a listener with such precise clarity that your hearer could repeat each phrase back to you word for word.

- You are encouraged to stick with that "audition piece" through many readings until you have made it your own.

- After you have mastered your piece, you can move on to another selection.

May your communication become clear and rewarding.

LESSON 3

FLOOR EXERCISES

In this lesson, you will take on six new exercises, all having to do with the floor. You will learn how to get down to the floor from your chair without getting hurt, but only after you have thought through how you will get back up into your chair from the floor. Nobody likes to get into anything they don't know how to get out of!

Thinking through a move in advance, figuring out the easiest, safest, and, yes, the cleverest way to accomplish that move, is called **movement strategy**. This is the first of the two important ideas in this lesson.

Once you have gotten down on the floor, you will ease down onto your side and end up on your back. From this position you will do two more spine-loosening exercises similar to the spine exercises in Lesson 1, but this time you will learn how to let gravity do most of the work. **Working with gravity** is the second important idea you will pick up in this lesson.

You will work with gravity to practice rolling over to your side and over onto your back. Finally you will get back onto your hands and knees and then climb back up into your chair. But first, we need to talk about making friends with the floor.

Fear of the Floor

Most people with PD regard the floor—whether it's the living room carpet, the ground, the sidewalk, or the street—as their enemy. "The ground just came up and whacked me," says one man. "I don't remember struggling, or losing my balance, or waving my arms. I'm just walking along, then—Wham! There's a bright flash when my head hit, and then there I am on the ground." A woman says, "I bent down to sweep some dust into a dustpan, and I just kept going straight down; I held on to the dustpan and it cut me over the eye. Seven stitches!" Another man says, "I closed the car door and started to step around the car, but my foot just didn't move. It was like it was stuck to the pavement. I made a grab for the door handle but missed. Down I went on my side; I bruised my hip and cut the palm of my hand. Hip still hurts five weeks later, but it's getting better." No wonder the floor seems like the enemy.

Take Patsy Metcalf, for example. Patsy had to depend on her husband Dick for quite a lot, which usually worked out all right because Dick was eminently dependable. She needed to place her walker a step ahead of herself, then take a step up to the walker, then place the walker ahead a step, and so forth. Using a railing she could pull herself up a flight of stairs hand over hand, while Dick carried the walker up and readied it for her at the top of the stairs.

Like all her classmates, Patsy dreaded falling, and for several good reasons. First and foremost she feared the broken hip that threatens everyone who is elderly. She had already dislocated a shoulder in a fall, which led to a lengthy and painful surgical reconstruction. She had no wish to repeat the hospital stay, the examinations, the X rays, or the pain medications.

Another thing she dreaded was falling in public. She hated drawing attention to herself, "making a scene" as she called it. Her classmates agreed, recounting stories of well-meaning people who tried to help, but only made things worse because they knew nothing about Parkinson's.

And if falling in public was bad, falling when alone was worse. Her classmate Oscar told of falling between the stove and the wall during a visit to the kitchen in the middle of the night. He was stuck in a position such that he could not back out or turn or get a grip on anything to pull himself up. He remained wedged there until his attendant arrived for the morning shift. "Funny now," he laughed, "but not very funny at the time."

Then Patsy started to tell us of "her real fear," but she got all choked up; her tears welled up and she couldn't speak out loud. We all moved closer to comfort her.

Finally we were able to put together the pieces of what she could say. What she feared most, her *real* fear, was that her husband, Dick, would get hurt trying to help her up. He had a long history of back problems, which he simply ignored when the need arose to lift his wife. "I try to stop him," she wept, "but Dick says, 'You have no choice, and that's the end of it.'"

It's a sad but simple fact: if you have Parkinson's disease, at some point, you are going to fall. Some people with PD fall once a year, some, once a day. Some people discover they have PD when they fall the first time; some people know they have PD and manage not to fall for ten years; but everybody falls. I am sorry, but that's the plain truth.

Little wonder that most people with Parkinson's regard the floor as their enemy. They fear what a fall to the floor may mean: injury, making a scene, being down and unable to get up, and causing injury to those who care for them. These fears are real, and we must have respect for them.

But no one wants to stop there. No one wants to be a prisoner of fear. If there is anything that can be done to make falls less likely to happen, or less damaging when they do happen, or less frightening when you are alone, or less dangerous to others, you want to know what it is.

Well, you're in luck, because that's exactly what this lesson is about: how to get as free as possible from these fears.

Facing Your Fear

Perhaps the first thing to recognize is that fear is your enemy, not the floor. Fear can tighten your muscles and joints, making your contact with the floor more jarring than it needs to be. Fear can keep you from thinking clearly about how to accomplish what needs to be done. Fear can hold you back from experimentation and even minimal risk-taking. Fearing loss of balance, you can overreact to a slight difficulty, stiffen your whole body in a panicky way, and lose your balance. Fear of falling is, in essence, a self-fulfilling prophecy: the fear can actually cause the fall. Make it clear to yourself: fear is the enemy.

You may have had your PD long enough to discover that your spouse's fear for you can be even more disabling than your own fear for yourself. The need to protect those we love burns brightly near the center of what most of us would call love. That protection, when powered by fear, can become fierce indeed. Fear can lead to overprotection, as your loved one anxiously hovers over your every effort, offering a constant stream of warnings and instructions, and impatiently "doing it for you" when you would rather do for yourself.

Fear is contagious. Your fear of your partner's fear will lead to impulsive actions on your part, actions that are not well thought through. Often, both of your fears will lead to irritable words and stubborn resistance that can make a difficult task nearly impossible. Your partner's fears must be taken into account along with your own. But they must not rule you, either of you.

You and your caregiver must confront fear step-by-step. Fear is like a tangled knot in a stiff rope: you need to take it apart and untie it one strand at a time. You need to separate out each possible danger, make a strategy to get around it, and refuse to let it hold you back.

Using Movement Strategies to Overcome Fear

Let's begin taking fear apart right now. Let's say that you might be afraid to get down on the floor because you won't be able to get back up. We'll do a *movement strategy session* that involves both you and your helper. Don't do the following movements; just read through them step-by-step, giving them your full attention:

- *You are going to get down on the floor. (You will be given instructions about how to get down when you are ready to actually do it.)*
- *You will not hurt yourself getting down.*
- *If your knees are very sensitive or the floor is too hard or too cold, you will be kneeling on a pad, or a blanket folded several times and laid out on the floor.*
- *You will be on your hands and knees.*
- *Your partner will move your chair around in front of you.*
- *You will crawl up very close to your chair.*
- *You will crawl forward until you can brace your upper body in the seat of the chair.*
- *You will lift one knee up far enough to put some weight on your foot, while still bending over into the chair.*
- *You will push your backside up in the air till you can put some weight on your other foot.*
- *You will still be bending over into the chair.*

- *Notice the physics of this move: your upper body will support itself on your forearms in the seat of the chair; therefore, your legs will only have to lift your lower body, only about half your full weight.*

- *Then you will stand the rest of the way up.*

- *You will turn around and sit back down in your chair.*

- *If turning is too difficult, your partner will move a chair behind you, and you will sit down right where you are.*

- *Home safe. Take a moment to celebrate!*

Now you and your partner go over this again, like the pilot and copilot checking off all the items on their "before takeoff" checklist. Your partner reads the instruction out loud, then you say it back:

Partner: "You are going to get down on the floor."

You: "I am going to get down on the floor."

Partner: "You will not hurt yourself getting down."

You: "I will not hurt myself getting down."

And so forth to the end of the list.

Now, read through and repeat back all the instructions before actually doing the exercise.

Exercises for the Transition from Floor to Chair

After you have finished reading through and repeating back all the instructions, you should go ahead and do the following exercise. Make sure the floor is clean and clear of obstacles. Put the pad down where it will be needed. Your helper may need to make these arrangements. The helper should try not to be "too helpful;" wait as long as you can before making a suggestion. Let the person doing the exercise work through the moves and learn from them. The first few times will be the most difficult.

EXERCISE 3.1
Creeping Down to the Floor

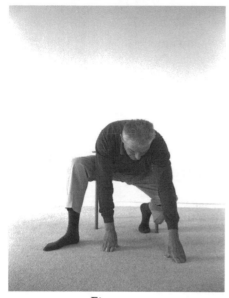

Figure 3.1

- Sit forward on the edge of your chair.
- Place your feet in a wide stance, knees wide open.
- Slide one foot back beside or under your chair, keeping your knees wide.
- With your elbows inside your knees, reach toward the floor as if you were going to "pick up the baby," but don't pick her up.
- Instead, place your fingertips down on the floor as far forward as you can manage.
- Put some weight on your hands. (See figure 3.1.)
- Increase the weight gradually.
- By now, your backside is already sliding off the front of your chair.
- Ease yourself down on one knee, without any noise.
- No Big Bumps! *Ease* your knee down.
- Put some weight on your knee and creep forward so your other knee will come down.
- You are now on your hands and knees.
- Rest for a moment, then do the next part.

EXERCISE 3.2
Climbing Up into Your Chair

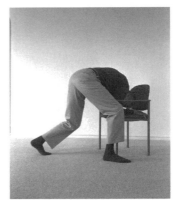

Figure 3.2a

- Crawl close to your chair, or pull the chair close to you. (If you cannot, your helper should *move the chair so it's directly in front of you.*)
- Place your elbows in the seat of the chair.
- Keep your head low, close to the seat of the chair. Lift one knee a little to the outside of the chair until you can put some weight on your foot.

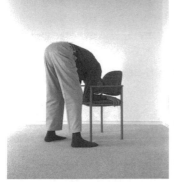

Figure 3.2b

- Once you have some weight on that leg, lift your backside way up. Bring the other knee up and get weight on both feet. (See figure 3.2a.)
- Your backside is now in the air, your elbows still in the seat of the chair. (See figure 3.2b.)
- Pause for a moment.

- Keep your head low till you are sure of your feet and till your breathing eases!
- Then use the arms of the chair to straighten up enough to turn and sit down. If you can't turn, your helper will place a chair behind you. (See figure 3.2c.)
- Sit down.
- You're home safe. Now really take a moment to celebrate!

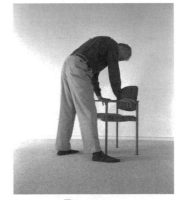

Figure 3.2c

You have gotten down to the floor and back up into your chair. Your helper has moved the chair to where you need it instead of trying to pick you up. You have thought through a movement strategy, considered the physics, and looked for the easiest, safest, and cleverest maneuver. You have good reason to celebrate. You are untangling the knot of fear one strand at a time.

Transitions

Getting down to the floor and back up into your chair are the first two of several **transitions** you will need to learn. Later I will take you through movement strategies for making the transition from sitting to standing, from standing to walking, from walking to lying down, and from walking to sitting. You will also learn many ways to make turns.

Transitions that people without PD take for granted can cause trouble for the person with PD. Starting and stopping, rising up and sitting down, changing directions when walking, reaching for something you've dropped, turning around in a small area, getting into a car, getting out of a car—all of these transitions can feel strange and unfriendly. The automatic weight shifts and shoulder turns no longer happen "automatically" for the person with PD; or they work fine at some times, and at other times, they unexpectedly balk, sputter, and halt.

Transitions are danger points. Injuries are most likely to happen during transitions: a person will struggle up out of a chair only to fall over the coffee table; a person standing at the sink doing dishes will begin to turn to put things away and will crash down, sometimes with the dishes; a person will get up from the bed in the dark and slide or tumble to the floor. Most people with PD install plenty of grab bars around the bathtub, the shower, and the toilet. You may not need them all the time, but you will almost certainly need them at least one time. And that one time is worth the cost.

You will need to practice transitions over and over till you remember to do them properly every time. Remember the carpenter's motto: "Plan three times, measure twice, cut once." You will often need to think through a move before you do it, and then do it one step at a time. Unfortunately, transitions do not become automatic; almost nothing becomes automatic for people with PD, except caution. You have to remember how to do it properly, every time.

Exercises for Working with Gravity

Now let's get back to making friends with the floor. Next you will learn four exercises that focus on working *with*, not *against*, gravity.

If you wear glasses, please take them off for the next set of exercises. They may get in your way. After getting down to the floor and lying on your back, you will be doing most of the exercises with your eyes closed, so you won't need your glasses anyway.

EXERCISE 3.3
Moving from Hands and Knees to Lying on Your Back

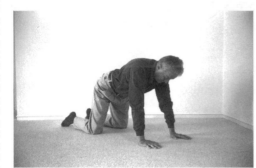

Figure 3.3a

- Go through the steps in exercise 3.1 to creep down to the floor and get to your hands and knees. (See figure 3.3a.)
- Now, starting from hands and knees . . .
- Move your LEFT hand farther to the LEFT.
- Shift all your weight on your LEFT hand.
- Move your RIGHT hand over next to your LEFT.
- Shift your weight onto both hands.

- *Ease* your left hip down to the floor. (No Bumps!)
- Now you are sitting on your LEFT hip still propped up by your hands. (See figure 3.3b.)
- Slide your hands forward until you are lying on your side.
- Make yourself comfortable. Make friends with the floor. Touch the floor with your hand. Feel textures of the rug or wood, notice the floor's temperature; remember, once you are down this far you can't fall any farther.

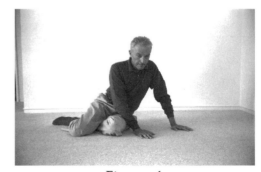

Figure 3.3b

- *Ease* your face down till the side of your face actually touches the surface of the floor. (See figure 3.3c.)

- Feel the floor with the side of your face.

- You are safe here for the moment.

- *Helper: Please place a pad behind the person if they need it to be comfortable, and be ready with a pillow.*

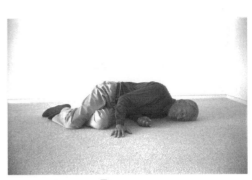

Figure 3.3c

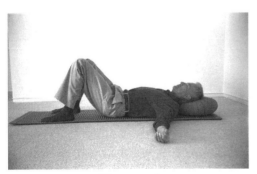

Figure 3.3d

- Roll over onto your back. (You will now be on the pad if you need one. Your helper can give you a pillow to put under your head if lying flat on your back is uncomfortable.)

- Settle down into the floor; get your weight even on both shoulders and on both sides of your bottom.

- Let your arms rest on the floor at your sides, hands palm up.

- Lift your knees up, placing your feet on the floor about a foot apart and as close to your backside as you can get them comfortably.

- We will call this position the Zero Position. (See figure 3.3d.)

You will do the following exercises starting from the Zero Position. After each exercise you will return to the Zero Position and get comfortable again.

This next group of exercises, *The Table with Two Legs* and the *Knees Fall* to both sides, are aimed at one of the most troublesome symptoms of PD. Most people with Parkinson's experience a stiffening of the muscles of the lower back and of the hips, perhaps as a result of uncertain balance reflexes. People with PD often walk as if they are walking on ice: short steps, eyes on the ground, body bent slightly forward, elbows close to the body, no arm swing. Such walking puts a strain on the lower back and hips, resulting in stiffness and often pain. These next exercises can begin to correct the problem.

Note to the helper: These three exercises flow from one to the next without hurry. Go slowly. If the person on the floor falls asleep, that's good. Wake them, and get them to yawn a few times. Then proceed.

EXERCISE 3.4
The Table with Two Legs

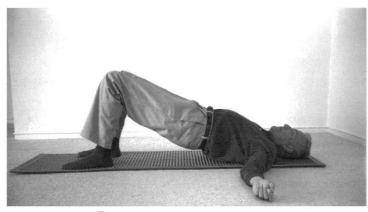

Figure 3.4a

- Start from the Zero Position.
- Close your eyes.
- Push down with your feet against the floor and pick your backside up to make a flat slope from your knees to your shoulders.
- You are now like a table that is missing two of its legs! That's why yoga teachers call this position "The Table with Two Legs." (See figure 3.4a.)
- (If this is hard to do at first, just lift your backside off the floor a few inches. You'll get better at this as time goes on.)
- Hold there for one minute.
- Breathe full tidal breaths while you hold.
- Notice that you don't need to push your arms down on the floor to hold your backside up.
- Relax your arms.
- Your weight is on your feet and your upper back.

Continued on next page

Exercise 3.4–Continued

- After one full minute, you'll feel glad it is time to come down.
- Lower your backside, but slowly, slowly.
- Let gravity pull you down.
- Make friends with gravity.
- Feel your tailbone touch the floor.
- Even after your backside is on the floor, you still have some more settling down to do *inside*.
- Feel your hips settling down.
- Let gravity do the work.
- Continue to let go of all the muscles in your hips and pelvis.
- You are back to the Zero Position.
- Now lift both knees up to your chest.
- Wrap your hands around your knees.
- Pull your knees toward your chest until it hurts good. (See figure 3.4b.)
- Breathe out a full exhale as you pull.
- Lower your feet back to the ground.
- Let everything settle down; let gravity do the work.
- Come to rest for a moment in the Zero Position.

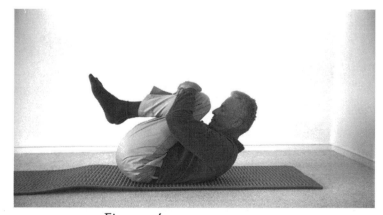

Figure 3.4b

EXERCISE 3.5
Knees Fall Left

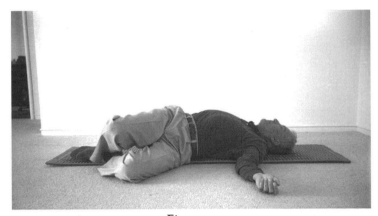

Figure 3.5

- Start from the Zero Position.

- Let your eyes close so you can pay attention to gravity and your sense of kinesthesia.

- Keep your eyes closed all through this exercise.

- Extend your arms out to both sides.

- Let gravity slowly pull both knees over to the LEFT. (See figure 3.5.)

- Keep your RIGHT hand on the ground.

- Pay attention to gravity as it slowly pulls both knees down as far as they will go.

- Enjoy the stretch in your waist and back.

- Notice you are in the same "spine rotation stretch" you did sitting up in your chair in Lesson 1, but this time you are not pulling yourself around, gravity is pulling you around.

- Now just lie there, eyes closed, and let gravity do the work.

- Breathe full breaths, in and out.

- Stay in this position for one minute.

- Then using as little effort as possible, bring your knees back up toward the Zero Position.

- Your legs may tremble a little as they come back; that won't hurt anything. Just notice the tremble and keep coming up to the Zero Position.

- Rest a moment. Get comfortable again.

- Do *The Table with Two Legs* for a moment.

- Pull your knees to your chest for a moment.

- Then lower your legs back to the Zero Position.

EXERCISE 3.6
Knees Fall Right

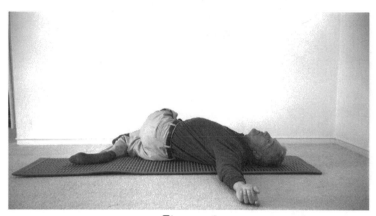

Figure 3.6

- Now do the same *Knees Fall* but this time to the RIGHT.

- Again, let gravity do the work.

- Take your time.

- Enjoy the "rotation stretch" on the other side of your waist. (See figure 3.6.)

- Breathe long breaths; feel your breath in your abdomen.

- After a full minute, come back up slowly to the Zero Position.

- Do *The Table with Two Legs* for a moment.

- Pull your knees to your chest for a moment.

- Settle back into the Zero Position.

Working with *Gravity*

Gravity is amazing when you stop to think about it. On the floor with your eyes closed, you can pay attention to the constant pull of gravity. By keeping your attention within the field of your kinesthesia, you will notice how gravity gives your muscles and bones a constant sense of weight. Gravity can also let you know about your movement as you notice your weight shifting from one support to another. And you may learn to marvel at how gravity gives you a sense of direction: "This way down!" it seems to say.

Gravity is always there. The stone cutters in the quarries of Carrera have for centuries hauled out huge blocks of translucent marble for sculptors and architects who adorned the palaces and cathedrals of Italy. The stone cutters used sleds drawn by ox teams for this dangerous work. Hardly a year went by without at least one man being killed by a block of marble in motion. Small wonder the cutters have a motto: "Weight never sleeps." Gravity can almost always tell you where you are if you pay attention to it.

In the following exercise, you will learn to use the weight of your legs falling to the side to help you roll over onto your side. And you can use the weight of your shoulders falling back to start your return roll onto your back. This is what is meant by working *with* gravity.

Remember to be incredibly lazy while you do these rolls. Gravity can't work for you if you insist on doing all the work yourself. Let yourself have several yawns before, during, and after each move. Take lots of time.

EXERCISE 3.7
Gravity Roll to Your Side and Back

· Start from the Zero Position.

· Close your eyes and feel your movements from the inside.

· Let gravity pull both knees to the LEFT.

· Leave your head at the center.

· When your knees are as far down to the LEFT as they will go, put your RIGHT hand on your chest.

· "Walk" your fingers from your chest to your LEFT shoulder, then down your LEFT arm, until they reach your LEFT hand.

· You will have rolled over onto your LEFT side, letting gravity do most of the work! (If you are using a pillow, shift it to be comfortable.)

· Notice the physics of this move: because your RIGHT hand was not extended out to your RIGHT like a wing, gravity was able to pull you over on your LEFT side.

· Now, reach back with your RIGHT hand out to your RIGHT again, until your shoulders are back on the ground.

· Now you are back to the "rotation stretch" position. (Seems familiar, doesn't it?)

· Let the weight of your shoulders opening out start the movement of your knees.

· Feel how gravity helps them come back up.

· Bring your knees up to the Zero Position.

· Open your eyes.

· When you are ready, roll over to your side using gravity to do the work.

· Come up onto your hands and knees.

· Move to your chair, or let your helper move your chair to you.

· Crawl up into your chair just as your did in the first exercise in this lesson.

· Celebrate for a moment!

So now you know what working with gravity can do. You can roll to either side and then back onto your back using gravity to make it easier. Instead of trying to roll to your side all at once, you let the bottom half of you go first. Then the weight of your falling knees makes it easier to roll your shoulders over to the side. Going the opposite way, you let your shoulders fall open onto your back first. Then the weight of your shoulders pulls your knees back toward the middle and there you are, on your back again. You are cooperating with gravity, instead of doing all the work yourself.

Summary

In this lesson you began to make friends with the floor:

- You got down to the floor and back up again without hurting yourself or your helper.

- You did this by making a **movement strategy** before you began, anticipating difficulties and solving them in advance, and then executing the strategy.

- In essence, you "planned three times, measured twice, and cut once."

Then you went down again to the floor and did three spine stretches lying on your back:

- You did *The Table with Two Legs* and *Knees Fall to the Left and Knees Fall to the Right*.

- You did this with your eyes closed so you could pay attention to gravity.

- Gravity kept you informed about weight, movement, and direction. Remember, "Weight never sleeps."

Then you used the power of gravity to roll over onto your side and back again. You have taken on the idea of **working with gravity** rather than doing all the work yourself.

By working with gravity, using movement strategy, and making friends with the floor by getting right down onto the floor for your workout, you have begun to untangle the knot of fear. Fear only makes a bad situation worse. Each day's workout should include time down on the floor.

In the next lesson, we will do more "floor work," as modern dancers call it. Like a dancer, you will become even better friends with the floor. When you are friends with the floor, instead of "falling," you will—like a dancer—"go to the floor!"

ON HANDS AND KNEES

As we said in the last lesson, sooner or later virtually every person with PD will fall. You began confronting your fear of falling by practicing getting back up from the floor with the help of a chair. You want to remember to use a chair to help you rather than putting your helper at risk by asking them to lift you unaided.

Injury and Immobility

Two other fears about falling haunt the person with Parkinson's disease: **injury** and **immobility**. These fears must be taken seriously. Falls can cause serious injuries; perhaps the most dreaded is a broken hip or pelvic bone, which can leave a person bedridden for months. Enforced inactivity brings with it the danger of muscle atrophy, joint stiffness, and respiratory infections. Add to that the potential for overworking your caregiver and running up medical expenses, and a broken hip becomes very scary indeed: For a person with PD prolonged confinement to a bed can be life-threatening, or at least life-shortening.

Other injuries include cuts requiring stitches, skinned knees, and scrapes along hands and forearms. Such injuries show up with distressing regularity at PD support-group meetings. Then there are sprains to ankles, knees, wrists, and elbows. Joint injuries usually take longer to heal than bruises and scrapes. Folks with PD need to keep ice packs handy in the freezer. They should also become experts on all the various pain relief and anti-inflammatory medications.

Last but not least in our list of fears about falling is immobility. Immobility when you are down can be a real problem. You may be down and possibly hurt, and you need to get to the phone. Or perhaps you've fallen in the bathroom in the middle of the night, and your caregiver is asleep in the other bedroom. Perhaps you live alone, and the weather is cold, and you need to get back to the bedroom, pull the blankets off the bed, and wrap yourself up on the floor until morning. Or a small grandchild left in your care is calling from another room and you can't get your legs to carry you. Even when you are not hurt, you may simply get tired of asking a caregiver to help you get up from the floor.

Every one of the above situations happened to people I have worked with. Immobility at floor level worries people with good reason.

Fred Collins, professor emeritus, would not allow Parkinson's disease to get in the way of his love for jazz. Parkinson's had caused his hands to curl inward and his fingers to seem knotted, but he had discovered—as many people with PD have—that his music could call his hands back into line. He could still play his keyboards, and he even took up an electronic wind instrument that fascinated him with its possibilities.

The best jazz club in town was a little over a mile from his house. Whenever Fred could, he would invite a few friends to accompany him to hear the fine artists as they passed through town. The friends would drive, and Fred would pay the cover charge. Sometimes nobody was available, the artist was just too good to miss, and Fred would go alone. He didn't trust his own driving at night, so he walked the little-over-a-mile from his house to the club, and after the show, when the club closed, he would walk back. "Good exercise," he called it when people worried about him.

Then one night, trouble. Most of Fred's route home went along well-lighted streets, but the last two blocks had only one streetlight between them, and the light from that was dimmed by the tall leafy trees lining the street. At one in the morning, and just twenty yards into his street, his shoe caught a crack in the sidewalk, and down he went to his hands and knees. When he gathered himself he found nothing bleeding or broken. But his medications seemed to have stopped working and he could not get back to his feet. He felt in his shirt pocket—impossible!—he had forgotten the little box that held his pills. No chance to take another pill and sit tight until he "came back on."

He tried pulling himself up with the help of a tree, but could not manage. He knew there would be nobody passing his way, and if anyone did pass they would most likely avoid him, thinking he was a drunk. He didn't think he could rouse his sleeping neighbors by calling out. He thought about crawling on hands and knees back to the main street with its lights and occasional passing cars, but decided against it. Instead, he set off for home—crawling on his hands and knees. He made his way in little five-yard spurts, after which he would rest a while, and then go at it again. It took him more than an hour to go the two blocks, but he made it.

When he told us about it a few days later, he also showed off his new knee pads with Velcro fasteners! "Don't leave home without 'em!" he chuckled.

The following exercises can help you **confront and overcome your fear of immobility**. You need to practice going to the floor again and again, until you become used to it. You need to rehearse letting yourself down to the floor a little at a time, until you become graceful. You need to practice getting back up over and over, until the strategy and the strength are there when you need them. And you need to crawl and scoot and crawl and scoot, not just to get around, but also to train your arms to bear your weight when you need them to absorb the shock of a fall.

Crawling and scooting will also help you **avoid injury** if you do fall. Bearing your weight (or half your weight, at least) on your arms actually strengthens your bones as well as your muscles. You need to strengthen your shoulders, wrists, and elbows to help you absorb the shock of landing.

Creep down to the floor in the careful way you learned in Lesson 3. Remember: No Bumps! Ease your knees down gracefully.

Now you are down and ready to begin. Remember the nicest thing about being down on the floor: you don't have to worry about falling, because you are already down.

Next come three pairs of floor exercises, all aimed at your upper body strength, flexibility, and safety when falling—or rather, safety when "going to the floor," as we like to say it. (There will be more discussion at the end of this lesson about how to change the way you think—and talk—about falling.)

Hands and Knees

This exercise requires you to put a good part of your weight on your hands. Remember to focus on your kinesthesia; keep your attention *inside* your body. You will feel the stretch mostly at your wrists, while the effort you will feel at your shoulders. As you bear your weight on your hands, arms, and shoulders, keep shifting around to get the most comfortable position. Concentrate on how your weight pushes your shoulders back. You can roll your shoulders forward and back to find the best support.

EXERCISE 4.1
Hands and Knees

· Place your hands palm down, well forward of your knees (think of "playing horsey" for a little one).
· Straighten and bend your elbows to find the most comfortable and secure support.
· Lean forward until a good part of your weight is on your hands.
· Rock your weight right and left a little to strengthen each shoulder.
· Lift one hand off the ground. Then lift the other.
· (If you are strong enough, lift your knees off the ground about two inches with both hands on the floor, of course.)
· Sit back until your weight is mostly on your knees.
· Lift one hand, shake it loose, put it down
· Lift the other hand, shake it loose, put it down.

There is good reason to work on the weight-bearing abilities of your shoulders: shoulder injuries are very common for people with Parkinson's disease. It is not unusual to see several people at a PD support-group meeting recovering from shoulder injuries. Either a shoulder gets pulled suddenly by grabbing at a handhold as the person falls, or a shoulder gets jammed back into its socket when a person lands with stiffly extended arms. Caregivers should also pay attention to the strength of their shoulders, because a sudden grab for a falling partner can injure a shoulder in a split second.

Always remember to take good care of yourself while you work out. You need to challenge yourself and go right to your limit so that you can improve, but you need to let yourself come to rest for a moment when you've reached that limit.

While putting your weight on your hands, don't put yourself through unnecessary pain. If your forearms feel they are getting too tired, try straightening your elbows a bit more. If your neck starts hurting from holding your head up, let your head drop forward and look back toward your knees; this will ease the neck strain. If your shoulders start hurting or feeling like they are going to give out on you, slip on down to the floor and come to rest for a moment on your elbows. *Only you* know when you need to ease up. Remember our motto: Easy does it; but do it.

Now you are ready for the alternate position, called the *Child's Pose*, which stretches and strengthens your shoulders.

EXERCISE 4.2
Child's Pose

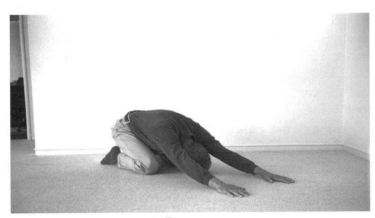

Figure 4.2

- Straighten your elbows and keep them as straight as you can.
- Sit back on your heels, or as close as you can get.
- Bow your forehead toward the floor between your outstretched arms.
- Let gravity do the work.
- Breathe three long full breaths in and out.
- This is called "the Child's Pose" in Yoga. (See figure 4.2.)
- Feel the really delicious stretch in your shoulders.
- Let gravity also work on your legs, knees, and feet.
- Feel the stretch around your knees, in your back, and in your calves.
- Go till it hurts good, then ease up.

Avoid unnecessary pain. Some people feel way too much pain in their feet as they start to sit back on them. You can place a small pillow between your feet and the floor; that should allow you to continue. Other people get foot cramps during *Child's Pose*. You may want to alternate between two ways of setting your feet when you drop back. In the first pose, point your toes back away from you so the tops of your feet rest on the floor; then, in the second pose, put your toes under your feet like a runner in the starting blocks. In both positions, ease your weight back slowly and stretch those muscles that want to cramp. They will gradually learn what you want them to do, and the cramps will stop.

Child's Pose should be thought of as a progressive exercise. The first few times you do it, you may not get very far. Don't be too hard on yourself, and don't give up. During each repetition (you will do three more in this next set), notice that you can go just a little bit farther back each time. After a month of daily workouts you will have progressed. You will be impressed at how much farther your shoulders will stretch and how much closer your backside gets to actually touching your heels.

Now you will do three alternations, from *Hands and Knees* to *Child's Pose*, with only one change per repetition: the position of your hands as they contact the floor. Each change of position will stretch and strengthen your hands, wrists, and forearms. You will see the need for all these different hand positions when you get to the crawling and scooting exercises.

EXERCISE 4.3
Change Shapes with Your Hands

- Come back to your hands and knees.
- Place your hands in *fists*, knuckles down. (See figure 4.3a.)
- Straighten and bend your elbows to find the most comfortable and secure support.
- Lean forward until a good part of your weight is on your hands.
- Rock your weight right and left a little to strengthen each shoulder.
- Lift one hand off the ground. Then lift the other.
- (If you are strong enough, lift your knees off the ground about two inches with both hands on the floor, of course.)

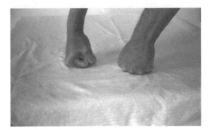

Figure 4.3a

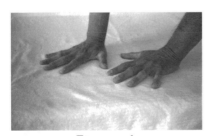

Figure 4.3b

- Sit back until your weight is mostly on your knees.
- Lift one hand, shake it loose, put it down *flat*. (See figure 4.3b.)
- Lift the other, shake it loose, put it down flat.
- Flatten your hands, straighten your arms, and drop back:
- *Child's Pose.*
- Come back to your hands and knees.

Continued on next page

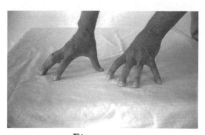

Figure 4.3c

- Place your hands on your *fingertips*. (See figure 4.3c.)
- Straighten and bend your elbows.
- Lean forward until a good part of your weight is on your hands.
- Rock your weight right and left a little.
- (If you can, lift your knees off the ground.)
- Sit back until your weight is mostly on your knees.
- Lift one hand, shake it loose, put it down flat.
- Lift the other hand, shake it loose, put it down flat.
- Flatten your hands, straighten your arms, and drop back:
- *Child's Pose.*
- Come back to your hands and knees.

- Rest your weight on your *second knuckles*; this is called "monkey knuckles." (See figure 4.3d.)
- Straighten and bend your elbows.
- Lean forward until a good part of your weight is on your hands.
- Rock your weight right and left a little.
- (If you can, lift your knees.)
- Sit back until your weight is mostly on your knees.
- Lift one hand, shake it loose, put it down
- Lift the other hand, shake it loose, put it down.
- Flatten your hands, straighten your arms, and drop back:
- *Child's Pose.*
- Come back to your hands and knees.

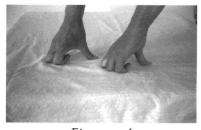

Figure 4.3d

Hip-Sit Exercises

The second pair of exercises again calls for weight-bearing by your arms. But now you will sit down on one hip, then return to your hands and knees; then you will sit down on the other hip, and then return to your hands and knees. This will improve your ability to lower yourself to the floor safely and to pick yourself back up to hands and knees. Getting down to your hip slowly allows gravity to stretch your lower back muscles in a way that hurts good.

These exercises continue your exploration of **movement strategy**. You will strategize the best way to sit down to your hip without any big bumps on your backside. Then you will *reverse* the strategy of the sit-down move to get back to your hands and knees with the least amount of effort. Remember that ease and power equal grace.

The second part of the movement, coming back to your hands and knees, will require some special attention to gracefulness. The most difficult part of getting to your hands and knees comes at the *first moment*—the first *inch* of lift—when you raise your hip from the floor. That first inch puts the most strain on your lower back and your shoulders. This exercise offers a movement strategy that will make getting up after a fall a whole lot easier and safer. Study that first moment of lift carefully; it does not seem "obvious" to most folks the first few times they try it. But once you learn how to do it, you'll wonder why you ever did it any other way.

Depending on your lower back strength and flexibility, you may do these exercises just once or several times. Don't overdo it. Start with one or two repetitions, then add more as you get more graceful. Rest frequently; focus on your kinesthesia; and give in to gravity: you want to work *with* it and not against it.

EXERCISE 4.4
Hip-Sit and Recovery

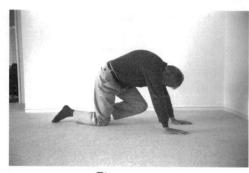

Figure 4.4a

- Come to your hands and knees.
- Pick up your LEFT knee.
- Notice that your weight is on both of your hands and your RIGHT knee.
- Move your LEFT knee around in a circle just off the ground.
- Set it down again. You are back on your hands and knees.

- Now you are ready for the next movement strategy: the Hip-Sit.
- Your hands will stay in the same place all through this next move.
- Move your LEFT knee up under your chest. (See figure 4.4a.)

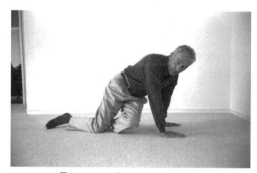

Figure 4.4b

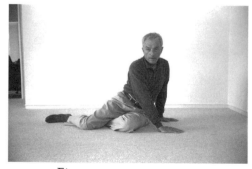

Figure 4.4c

- Slide your LEFT knee *across* your body. (See figure 4.4b.)
- Lower your LEFT hip slowly down to the ground. (See figure 4.4c.)

- Just before your hip reaches the ground, STOP for a moment and take a mental snapshot of where you are: "Your weight rests on your hands and your RIGHT knee, while your LEFT leg (hip *and* knee) is parallel to and just off the floor." You'll need to remember this position in the next "reversal" exercise.

- Sit on your hip and come to rest for a moment.

- This is the Hip-Sit position. (See figure 4.4d.)

- Do a few mini-pushups to get comfortable in this position.

- Now you will do that whole move in reverse.

- Shift your weight forward onto your hands.

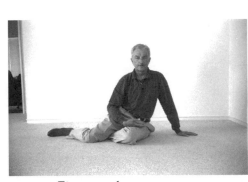

Figure 4.4d

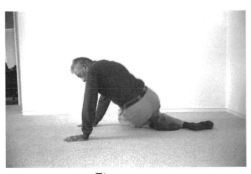

Figure 4.4e

- Return your weight to your hands and your RIGHT knee.

- Double check that: two hands and RIGHT knee.

- Raise your LEFT leg (hip and knee) a little up from the ground. (See figure 4.4e.)

- Remember your mental snapshot from the last exercise? "Your weight rests on your hands and your RIGHT knee, while your LEFT leg (hip *and* knee) is parallel to and just off the floor." That's where you should be. If you are not there, sit back down on your hip and try it again. If you don't get this the first few times, don't worry. Eventually you will.

- Bring your LEFT knee back from across your body.

Continued on next page

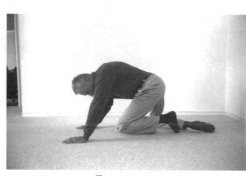

Figure 4.4f

- Move your LEFT knee back under you. (See figure 4.4f.)
- There you are back at your hands and knees position. (See figure 4.4g.)
- Come to rest for a moment.
- The second part of this exercise simply mirrors the above, coming down on the *RIGHT* hip.
- Start from your hands and knees.

- Lift your RIGHT knee, move it in circles, move it all around.
- Bring your RIGHT knee forward under your chest.
- Slide your RIGHT knee across your body.
- Settle down into your RIGHT Hip-Sit. (No Bumps!)
- Reverse the process as before:
- Shift weight to your hands and LEFT knee.
- Double check that: two hands and LEFT knee.
- Raise your RIGHT leg (hip *and* knee) a little up from the ground.
- Bring your RIGHT knee back from across your body.
- Move your RIGHT knee back under you.
- There you are, back at your hands and knees position.
- Come to rest for a moment.

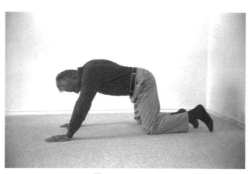

Figure 4.4g

You should repeat the movements until they feel natural. You will notice that both movements, down to the Hip-Sit and back up to your hands and knees, are very efficient. That's because they are modeled on the movements of a cat. Next time you get a chance to observe a cat, you can check this out.

Your performance of these moves depends on the *Spine Rotation* stretch you started practicing back in Lesson 1. You also practiced that same stretch in *Knees Fall* in Lesson 3. You will get better at your lumbar rotation as you become more flexible. Again, let gravity do most of the work. Learn to enjoy the stretching sensation around your waist as you settle down into the Hip-Sit position.

Practicing the *Hip-Sit and Recovery* exercises will prepare you for two possible problems you may encounter after a fall. First, when you fall to the side, you are most likely to land in exactly this Hip-Sit position. You want your shoulders and hands to be strong and flexible (not stiff!) when they break your fall. You want your hip and thigh to be accustomed to contact with the floor.

Second, getting back onto your hands and knees can be difficult, especially if you are excited, as you probably will be when you have an unintended fall. You want to know how to get back up in the easiest way possible. You want your waist to be strong and flexible enough to make that lift-up-your-hip-and-slide-your-knee-back-under-you move that gets you back in business, back on your hands and knees.

Crawling and Scooting Exercises

In the third and last pair of exercises, you will alternate two modes of floor-level locomotion: crawling and scooting on your backside. Not very dignified, probably, but what the heck, it gets you there! And that's what you need to overcome your fear of a fall: the knowledge that you can get where you want to go one way or another.

EXERCISE 4.5
Crawling and Scooting

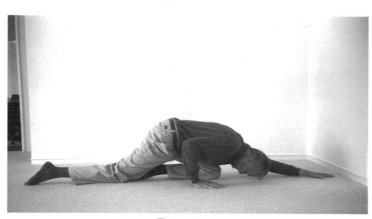

Figure 4.5a

- Come to your hands and knees.
- Go for a crawl around the room.
- (Are your hands taking just tiny little steps? Many people with Parkinson's disease will be familiar with these tiny steps. If you take long steps with your hands, your knees will also take long steps.)
- Take nice long "steps" with your hands. (See figure 4.5a.)
- You will probably notice that your wrists get tired first. Change your hand position frequently: from flat, to fists, to fingertips, to "monkey knuckles." This will protect your wrists from fatigue.
- Keep on crawling and exploring the room.
- Imagine you are a cat, or an elephant, or some other animal. Yawn. Growl. Scratch. Have fun.
- Keep changing the position of your hands to ease the tiredness in your wrists.
- Use flat hands for a while, then fists, then fingertips, then monkey knuckles. (See the figures in exercise 4.3.)
- Now, sit down to one hip, in the manner you just learned.

- Shift over to sit on your bottom.
- Push down with your hands and feet and lift your bottom off the floor. (See figure 4.5b.)
- Now scoot it along.
- Sit down.
- Move your hands and feet.
- Lift bottom, scoot along, move your hands and feet, scoot along, and so on.
- Scoot around the room.
- Try going forward, backward, to the side, to the other side.
- Change your hand position frequently: flat, fists, fingertips, monkey knuckles. This will protect your wrists from fatigue. Your wrists will get stronger with practice.
- Now you are ready to finish.
- Come to the Hip/Sit position.
- Shift onto your hands and knees in the manner you learned.
- Crawl to your chair.
- Pull yourself up into the chair. (Be sure to do it the way you practiced before!)

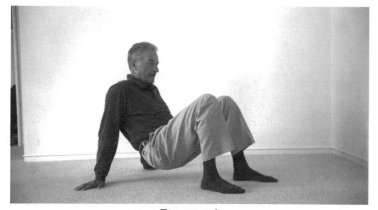

Figure 4.5b

Most people with Parkinson's know they must stay active. They find a way around their limitations in order to continue doing what needs to be done. They want to be useful. Doing something useful can be the best remedy for the blues, and dealing with a chronic illness can definitely bring on the blues. So take every opportunity to integrate your new movement strategies into your exercise routine and into your daily life.

Melvin Gilbert's wife worked a full-time job and then came home to a full set of domestic duties. Melvin wanted to take over some of the chores. He tried to carry the laundry basket to the basement on washday and landed on top of the basket at the bottom of the stairs, so he had to settle for being the one to fold the laundry. To remind himself of how to move about on the floor, he'd set the basket of clean laundry on the floor by the couch, and do the folding on his knees. This allowed him to integrate his exercises into his daily routine!

"Big Joe" Caldwell needed to babyproof his kitchen and family room so he could take care of his twin granddaughters while his daughter ran errands. By crawling around the house he figured out many areas he needed to make safe for the girls. He also found he could manage them fairly well by sitting on the floor with them. "They think I'm just a really big toy they can climb all over," he says, not really complaining. Being down at their level was a great way to incorporate these exercises into his life.

Look around the house for ways to work or play down at floor level. That will accustom you to getting down to the floor, moving around, and getting back up. There's an old joke about getting old you may have heard: You know you're getting old if, when you stoop down to tie your shoes, you look around to see if there's anything else you can do while you're down there.

Summary

In this workout session you came down to your hands and knees to do three pairs of shoulder-strengthening exercises:

- You used four different hand positions as you shifted your weight forward onto your hands and arms. You alternated these four weight-bearing efforts with a drop back into a shoulder stretching *Child's Pose*.

- You practiced dropping into the Hip-Sit position by bringing one knee forward and across. After each sit you raised yourself again to your hands and knees using the same movement strategy in reverse.

- You finished the exercise set by alternating between crawling and scooting as you explored your environment. You remembered to keep changing your hand position to ease the strain on your wrists.

The following are some other ways to overcome your fear of the floor:

- Tell yourself that you can change "falling" into "going to the floor."

- Rehearse "going to the floor" again and again and you will become more graceful at it.

- Practice coming back to your hands and knees, gracefully, strategically.

- Once back to your hands and knees, convince yourself that you can crawl or scoot to safety again.

- You already know how to creep back up into a chair.

If you start calling these scary events "going to the floor" instead of "falling," then, maybe, when that time comes when you do start into a fall, things will feel so familiar that on the way down you will think of it as "going to the floor"!

Happy landings!

LEG STRETCHES

In this lesson we will discuss the balance problem called **retropulsion** and its close cousin **propulsion.** Many people with Parkinson's disease have difficulty standing up from a chair without tumbling backward; that's retropulsion. Others at times will make a series of accelerating little forward steps, a kind of stuttering step; that's propulsion. Both problems originate in malfunctions of your **postural reflexes.**

Your new workout exercises will focus on these problems. First will come a series of stretches aimed at your hamstrings, calves, ankles, and feet. Then you will practice a new movement strategy for standing up from a chair without losing your balance. You will learn two versions of this movement strategy, one for very unsteady people, the other for more confident folks.

First, a story.

Bill Parker had more courage sometimes than good sense, but at seventy-two nobody was about to change him. He was, shall we say, just a little bit competitive. Out for a walk one day, he saw a few local runners in expensive sweatsuits turn onto the steepest hill in town and charge right up it. This is the kind of hill where they post signs saying "Trucks Use Low Gears" on the downslope. He figured that if those yuppies could *run* up that hill, why then he could surely *walk* up that hill. He was about a third of the way up when, naturally enough, he stopped to catch his breath. Unfortunately, he was still facing uphill. As soon as he stopped, he seemed to tilt backward. One little step backward to catch himself, then several more little steps in rapid succession . . . and he knew he was in big trouble.

Fortunately for him, he did not land on the concrete as he expected, but instead sailed over backward and wound up spread-eagled in some lady's hedge. The hedge cushioned his fall, but now there was no way he could get himself back on his feet. So he just lay there quietly, listening for the sound of somebody passing.

Cars passed. Birds sang. Finally, he heard a dog sniffing about, and he called out, "Hello there, can you give me a hand?" This really scared the dog, but the dog's owner helped him out. Bill left a note on the hedge lady's door with his phone number and an offer to pay for the damage, but she never called.

Postural Reflexes

Many people with PD have Bill's "backward-stepping" problem; it is called *retropulsion.* They will stand up from a chair only to tumble suddenly backward (hopefully right back down into the chair). Or they will start to step back from a counter, or to step out of some other person's path, or to reach up to a high shelf, and suddenly they take several short steps backward trying to catch their balance. Sometimes they manage, sometimes only a wall stops them, sometimes they have to turn and catch themselves on some handhold. Sometimes they go to the floor.

Propulsion, a similar problem but in the forward direction, usually develops later in a person's PD career than retropulsion. A standing person will suddenly lean forward, then take many small steps forward, without really catching their balance. One of our group members calls it "stotting"—a combination of stuttering and trotting.

Whatever you want to call it, the problem shows some malfunction in your *postural reflexes.* Postural reflexes do not function properly in people with Parkinson's. When your neurologist tested you for Parkinson's, you may remember that he or she came around behind you and without much warning jerked you backward at your shoulders. You may have been startled, but of course the doctor kept you from falling over backward. That was a test of your postural reflexes. If your postural reflexes are working well your body makes a little jerk and you're back in balance. If the doctor had to catch you to keep you from falling backward, you flunked the test.

There are several **postural reflexes** throughout your body that make automatic adjustments to keep your balance and to protect your joints from injury. You've seen people standing up in a crowded bus all make that little jerk when the bus starts or stops suddenly. No matter which way each person is standing—facing forward, backward, or sideways, their amazing postural reflexes make that little jerk and they keep their balance. People with PD should not stand up on buses!

How do postural reflexes work? Let's take an example. One postural reflex adjusts your ankle every time you take a step. There are nerve endings in the soles of your feet that detect the surface of the ground as you bring your foot down. The bottom of your foot can detect regularities and irregularities. Amazing when you think about it. The sole of your foot can tell sand from gravel from concrete from grass from ice from asphalt and so on. It can detect tilt in any direction. It can sense if the ground has a convex curve or a concave curve, and it can sense if the ground is flat. It can measure the shape of support under your foot—as on a tightrope or a ladder rung—and tell where there is no support—as for example in all the open air around the tightrope or the ladder rung.

All that information travels through nerves up through your legs to a special nerve center near the base of your spine. Now here is where the "reflex" comes in. Usually, information from your senses is sent on up your spine to your brain for processing, but not this surface-under-my-feet information. Instead, that special nerve center near the base of your spine makes a *reflex* judgment about what to do to keep your balance and to protect your ankle from injury. The nerve center then sends immediate action messages to your calf muscles that adjust the tensions around your ankle to correct your balance and avoid injury to your ankle and knee joints.

This reflex adjustment happens very fast because it needs to happen very fast. Think about how we must have evolved our upright walking and running posture. We would have to be able to chase down game or escape from predators across uneven terrain. No time to look at the ground; we have to keep our eyes fixed on our quarry or on the moves of whatever is chasing us. If you can remember running across open fields or through woodlands with the breakneck bravado of childhood, you can remember stepping on stones and tussocks of grass, the unexpected cave in of an underground burrow, or the sudden slipperiness of a wet patch of leaves. Your body has to make an adjustment between the time when the foot touches the irregularity and the time you bring your full weight onto the foot: a tiny fraction of a second. No time to consult with the conscious mind; therefore our marvelous body has evolved this ankle-adjusting reflex.

Now the bad news. Postural reflexes are compromised by Parkinson's disease. In the early stages of the disease they work most of the time and malfunction occasionally. As the disease progresses, they become more and more unreliable. Rigidity causes most of the problem. People with Parkinson's begin to stand and walk more cautiously. Like people walking on ice, they expect difficulty keeping their footing. That extra caution adds tension to already rigid muscles and joints, and compounds the problem. Tight muscles are less responsive to postural reflex signals than are relaxed and flexible muscles.

When I first began working with people with Parkinson's, I watched their characteristic cautious way of walking and I thought, "Where have I seen that way of walking before?" Then I remembered. I myself had walked that way for two weeks in 1954, my first two weeks at sea with the United States Navy! Handhold to handhold, from dinner tray to leaning over the side, what a misery for this farm boy! Finally I got what they called my "sea legs," and then I could saunter down a pitching deck with the best of them.

Overcoming Postural Reflex Problems

What can be done about retropulsion, propulsion, and those unreliable postural reflexes? First, you need to stretch your hamstrings, calves, ankles, and feet. You want to make them flexible, so they can move quickly when a postural reflex signal asks them to. Second, you need to develop a movement strategy to go from sitting to standing safely. You want to avoid that moment of unsteadiness that plops you back into your chair. Third, you need to challenge your postural reflexes by practicing exercises and games in a safe environment (not by climbing a "Trucks-Use-Low-Gears" hill on impulse!). Challenging your reflexes in a safe way makes them lively, keeps your muscles and joints flexible, and makes you more confident of your abilities. Confidence reduces your tension and thus reduces your difficulty balancing.

We will handle the first two, the stretches and the standing up strategy, in the remainder of this lesson. We will take up the third, the balance challenges, in succeeding lessons.

You are already on your way. The exercises you have been doing in the earlier lessons have already stretched key muscle groups, loosened up the most rigid joints, and sensitized nerve endings to be ready for action—"postural reflex" action.

Your spine can bend, twist, and drop a bit more than before you began daily work-outs. Your shoulders and hips can move in opposite directions. The bottoms of your feet have been sensitized by that tennis ball. Your ankles have been rocking and rolling keeping on top of the ball. Your hands, wrists, and arms are more flexible and stronger, ready to do their part. And your hips have been pushed outward, rolled left and right, stretched, and tucked under—preparing them to "make that little jerk" that saves your balance.

But enough of the pep talk, let's get on with the new exercises.

Leg Stretches

First, you will work with your legs. Your hamstrings need to be stretched, your calves need to be stretched, and your ankles and toes need to be stretched. We will let gravity do all the work. Your part is to assume the positions and endure the pain ... I mean, the "hurts good." These exercises hurt a bit, there's no getting around that. Do them slowly, steadily, relentlessly; do not hurry, do not bounce, and keep yourself calm and safe. Practice your groaning! Make your groans very convincing! Easy does it; but do it.

EXERCISE 5.1
Hamstring Stretch

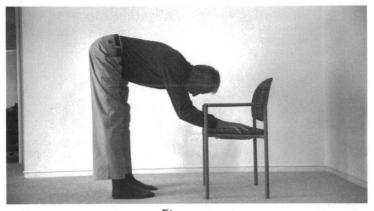

Figure 5.1

- Come up to standing.
- Turn and face your "sturdy chair with arms."
- Set your feet about shoulder width apart.
- Bend forward and place your hands on the arms of the chair.
- Keep your knees straight.
- Move your feet back a bit.
- Wiggle your backside to make your back flat.
- Now move your fingertips to the seat of the chair.
- Support yourself on just your fingertips.
- Keep your knees straight.
- You will feel a stretch in your hamstring. Ease into that stretch, try to enjoy it, let it hurt good.
- Move your hands back up to the arms of the chair.
- Rest a bit, complain a little (complaining is good for the voice).
- Now move your hands again to the seat of the chair.
- Support yourself on your "monkey knuckles."
- Let your back be flat.
- Keep your knees straight.
- Wag your tail a little. Yawn.
- Let gravity do the stretch, ease into it, keep breathing.
- Come back to the arms of the chair, rest, complain.
- Move your hands to the seat of the chair.
- Support yourself on your flat palms. (See figure 5.1.)
- If you can already do that, try supporting yourself on your elbows! Now *that* is a hamstring stretch!

If you can get your elbows to touch the seat of the chair with your legs straight, you may be able to touch your toes! Try pushing the chair a little farther away from you to see if you can reach down that far. Even if your are two or four or six inches away, that's fine. Now you have something to measure the progress of your hamstring stretches. If you do these stretches during your daily workout, you may indeed be able to touch your toes in time. That should be your goal.

EXERCISE 5.2
Calf Stretch

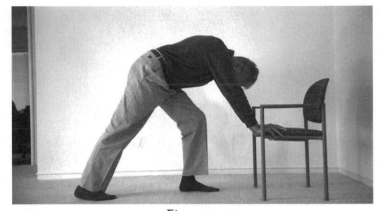

Figure 5.2

- Brace you hands on the arms of the chair.
- Move your RIGHT leg back at least two feet.
- Put the ball of your RIGHT foot down.
- Straighten your RIGHT knee.
- Now slowly press your RIGHT heel down to the floor. (See figure 5.2.)
- Keep your toes, knee, and heel lined up, pointing straight ahead toward your chair.

- Ease up a moment.
- Move the RIGHT leg farther back.
- Again, slowly press your heel to the floor.
- Let gravity do the work. Breathe long full breaths.
- Bring your RIGHT leg forward.
- Come to rest for a moment.
- Now, do the LEFT leg.

EXERCISE 5.3
Ankle and Toe Stretch

- Kneel down facing your chair.
- Point your toes *back and away* from you.
- The tops of your feet should be in contact with the floor.
- (If the tops of your feet hurt too much, place a small pillow between your feet and the floor.)
- Slowly sit back on your heels. (See figure 5.3a.)

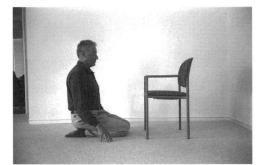

Figure 5.3a

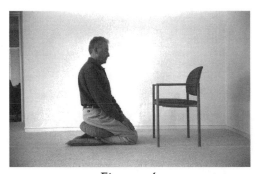

Figure 5.3b

- Use your hands on the floor to slow your descent.
- Do not go past the "hurts good" point.
- If you can, sit all the way down on your heels with your hands in your lap.
- (If you cannot sit all the way down, try placing a fat pillow between your backside and your ankles. [See figure 5.3b.])

Continued on next page

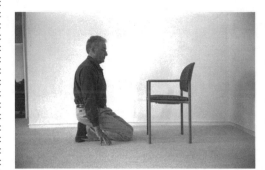

Figure 5.3c

- Sit upright over your heels with your hands in your lap.
- If you can yawn in spite of the "hurts good," you may give yourself a gold star.
- Now lean forward into the chair.
- Tuck your toes *under* you.
- Again, slowly sit back over your feet. (See figure 5.3c.)

- This will stretch your toes like crazy.
- If you can, sit all the way down on your heels, with your hands in your lap. (See figure 5.3d.)
- Let gravity do the work.
- Breathe full. Complain out loud.
- This completes the toe and ankle stretch.

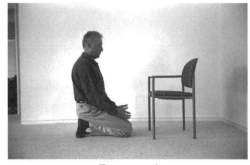

Figure 5.3d

Movement Strategies for Standing Up from a Chair

Now for the retropulsion. Let's work on the movement strategy for moving from sitting to standing without falling backward suddenly. This skill can be developed, but you have to remember to use it. Once you know how to do it, you can say good-bye to tumbling back into your chair.

The movement strategy for standing up is similar to the one you used to creep up into a chair from your hands and knees. You lower your top half, lift your bottom half, then lift your top half. That way your legs only need to lift about half your weight in the first part of the move. Once you have your legs under you, all you have to do is uncurl your spine, and your top half comes right on up. Very economical.

I am going to give you two versions of this exercise, both are elegant and graceful. The first version is for people with less strength in their legs or less confidence in their balance. The second version should be used by people who have reasonable confidence in both their legs and their balance. Here's how it is done:

EXERCISE 5.4
Standing Up from a Chair (First Version)

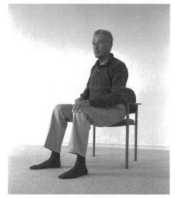

Figure 5.4a

- Sit forward on the edge of your chair.
- Put both knees over to the RIGHT a full 45 degrees.
- Separate your feet at least twelve inches. (See figure 5.4a.)
- Put your RIGHT foot forward.

- Put your LEFT foot back, opened out a little. (See figure 5.4b.)
- Put your RIGHT hand on the arm of the chair.
- Put your LEFT hand on your left knee.

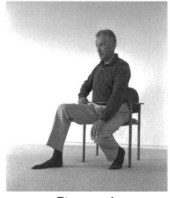

Figure 5.4b

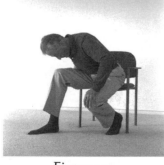

Figure 5.4c

- Bend forward as if you mean to kiss your RIGHT knee. (See figure 5.4c.)
- The farther forward you bend the better.
- Keep looking back between your knees.

- Lift your backside off the chair. (See figure 5.4d.)
- Straighten your legs as much as you can.
- You should still be head down, looking back between your knees.

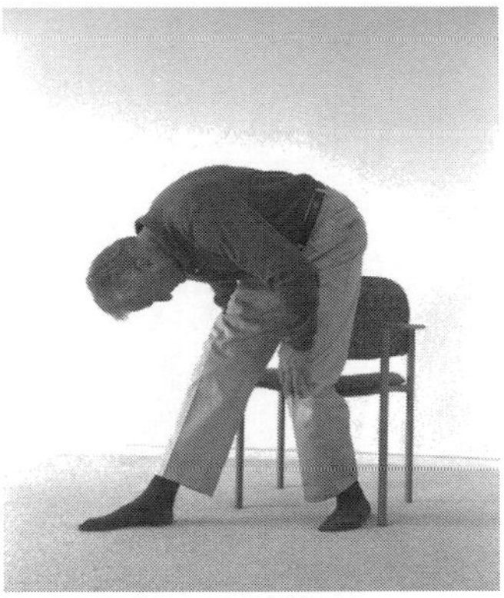

Figure 5.4d

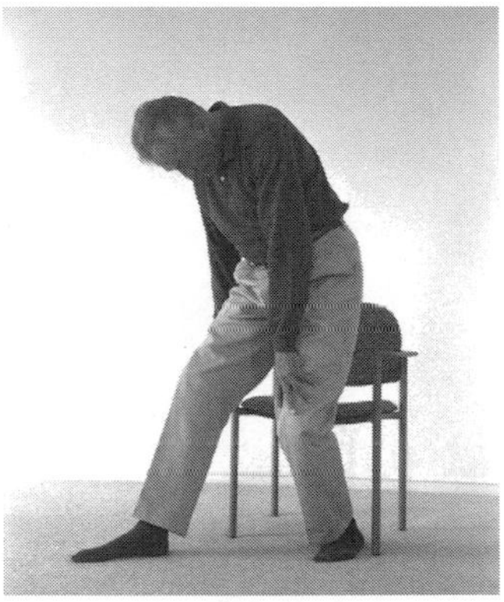

- Now uncurl your spine, like you're unrolling a spool of ribbon. Bring your upper body up to standing. (See figure 5.4e.)
- Look at your navel all the way up.

Figure 5.4e

- Lift your head. (Your head should be the last part to come up.)
- There you are, standing, right leg a little ahead of the LEFT. (See figure 5.4f.)
- Congratulations!

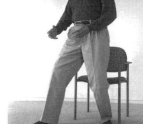

Figure 5.4f

Now here is the second version. You will stand up without holding on to the arms of the chair or bracing your hands on your knees. You may recognize several elements of this movement strategy from your exercise routines in earlier lessons.

EXERCISE 5.5
Standing Up from a Chair (Second Version)

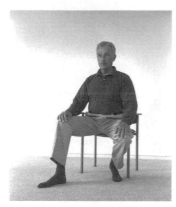

Figure 5.5a

· Sit forward on the edge of your chair.
· Move one foot back under the edge of the chair. (See figure 5.5a.)
· Set both feet pointing forward.
· Reach down with both arms inside your knees. (You may remember this as "reach down to pick up the baby.")

· Reach out as far as you can along the floor. (See figure 5.5b.)
· Let your backside come forward out of the chair (it probably has already done so!).

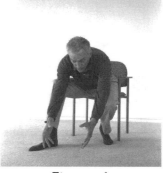

Figure 5.5b

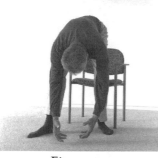

Figure 5.5c

· Now put all your weight on your feet.
· Push your backside up a bit to get ready.
· Pick up the imaginary baby. (See figure 5.5c.)
· Start standing up.

· Keep the baby close enough to kiss her all the way up. (See figure 5.5d.) This will keep your head tucked until you are upright.

· Uncurl your spine, like a roll of ribbon unrolling up to the moon.

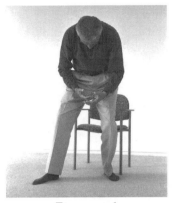

Figure 5.5d

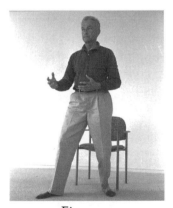

Figure 5.5e

· Come all the way up to standing.

· Let your head be the last part to come up.

· There you are, standing, one foot forward, one foot back. (See figure 5.5e.)

· Congratulations!

Now try the old way of standing up. Sit forward, keep your feet side by side, put your hands on the arms of the chair, and try standing up while keeping your head way up on top of everything. You'll notice how much more effort you need. You may even notice that there's a moment when you have to sort of jump—or at least push off a bit extra—to go from supporting yourself with your hands to being just on two feet. That little jump is what you want to avoid. That's the moment when your postural reflex should set you right, but cannot, because, as we said before, postural reflexes don't function reliably for people with Parkinson's.

Now practice the new movement strategy again, either the first or second version. Sit forward, set one foot forward and one foot back, bend down to pick up the baby, push your backside up, uncurl your spine, and you are up. Notice the physics, notice the flow of the movement. No little jump needed. And remember: No little jump means there is no need for your postural reflexes to keep you balanced. *You are completely in balance all through the movement!*

Summary

This lesson covered two balance problems, **retropulsion** and **propulsion.** The first involves stumbling backward and the second involves stumbling forward. Both problems appear in PD due to slow responses to **postural reflex** signals:

- Postural reflexes are compromised in people with PD, due largely to increased rigidity in the person's legs.
- Regular practice of a set of stretching exercises for hamstrings, calves, ankles, and feet can make leg muscles and joints more flexible and responsive.
- Since retropulsion makes standing up from a chair particularly difficult, it makes sense to develop and practice a **movement strategy** for standing up safely.

The lesson closes with two movement strategies for standing up from a chair safely, one for people who need to be very careful, another for stronger people.

In the following lessons we will continue our work with balance problems. You can expect exercises and games that challenge your postural reflexes without putting you in danger of falling. "Developing skills through challenges in a safe setting" is a good working definition of "play." And that is precisely what you will be doing throughout this book: using **play** to develop improved skills for coping with Parkinson's disease.

GOING TO THE FLOOR

People who have had PD for a long time will tell you, "Learn to fall long before you need to learn to fall." This advice makes sense when you consider that in the early years of your PD career you may still have a good portion of your strength and flexibility. Once you have suffered an injury in a fall, you may be so wary of falling again that you tighten up and make things more difficult to learn than they need to be. You need to reduce your *fear* of falling. And as we discussed in our previous lesson, the best way to reduce your fear is to learn a movement strategy and walk yourself right through it, one step at a time.

Learning to Go to the Floor

This lesson will teach you to **go to the floor on purpose**. You will practice going down to the floor from a standing position with all your attention focused on how you are doing it. You will stay completely aware of every part of the movement. You will figure out how to go down safely and, would you believe it, gracefully.

Your floor work and crawling exercises have already prepared you to go to the floor safely. Putting weight on your arms, wrists, and hands has made them stronger and more flexible. Your shoulders have gotten used to supporting your weight during your earlier crawling exercises. The *Hip-Sit* exercises have prepared your lower back for the necessary twist. You have gotten used to sitting on your hip. You are ready to go to the floor safely.

You can start right from where you left off in the last lesson, standing up from your chair with one foot ahead of the other and with your weight on both feet. Then you will go through the steps that get you down to the floor safely.

EXERCISE 6.1
Going to the Floor to the Right Side

- Put your LEFT foot forward and out (at about 20 degrees from center).
- Hold an imaginary baby.
- Bend your knees till your hands are closer to the floor (enough to put the baby down gently).
- Put both hands over to the RIGHT and down toward the floor.
- Put the baby down.
- Reach beyond the baby.
- Put some weight on your hands. (See figure 6.1a.)

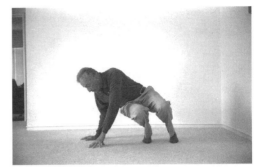

Figure 6.1a

- Bring your RIGHT hip down to the Hip-Sit position. (See figure 6.1b.)
- Come to rest for a moment.
- Move to hands and knees in the manner you learned.
- Crawl to a chair.
- Use your chair to help you come to standing in the manner you learned in Lesson 3.
- Remember, your backside comes up first, then your upper body uncurls to standing.
- (If you need to sit and rest, do so. If not, just come to standing and go on to the next exercise. Easy does it; but do it.)
- If you need to rest, rest as long as you need.

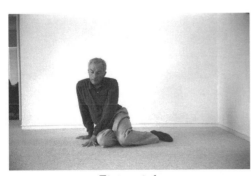

Figure 6.1b

EXERCISE 6.2
Going to the Floor to the Left Side

- Place your RIGHT foot forward and out (at about 20 degrees).

- Hold an imaginary baby.

- Bend your knees enough to put the baby down gently.

- Put both hands over to the LEFT and down toward the floor.

- Put the baby down.

- Reach beyond the baby.

- Put some weight on your hands.

- Bring your LEFT hip down to the Hip-Sit position.

- Come to a rest for a moment.

- Move to hands and knees in the manner you learned.

- Crawl to your chair.

- Use your chair to help you come to standing in the manner you learned in Lesson 3.

- Remember, your backside comes up first, then your upper body uncurls to standing.

- (If you need to sit and rest, do so. If not, just come to standing and go on to the next exercise.)

- Easy does it; but do it.

EXERCISE 6.3
Going to the Floor Forward

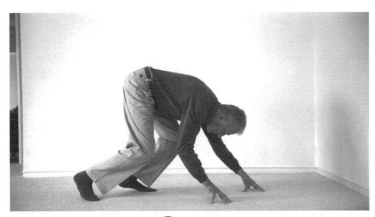

Figure 6.3

- Start from a standing position.
- Hold an imaginary baby.
- Bend your knees.
- Curl your spine forward till you can put the imaginary baby down on the floor. Gently; no jerks.
- Then reach out forward along the floor with your hands.
- Set one hand short and one hand long.
- Put some weight on your hands. (See figure 6.3.)
- Lower your knees to the floor without any bumps.

- You may need to take a step forward with your hands.
- Come to rest for a moment on your hands and knees.
- Crawl to your chair.
- Use your chair to help you come to standing in the manner you learned in Lesson 3.
- Remember, your backside comes up first, then your upper body uncurls to standing.
- (If you need to sit and rest, do so. If not, just come to standing and go on to the next exercise.)
- Easy does it; but do it.

You have been practicing going to the floor forward, to the right, and to the left. You have not been "falling"; you have been "going to the floor" in very slow motion, taking care to protect yourself all along. By putting the baby down on the floor near your feet, you lower your center of gravity and bring your arms into position to reach the floor first. That way your arms can begin to take some of your weight before your knees or your hip reaches the floor. This strategy spreads the shock around to several points of contact, lessening the impact on each one. The motto is the same as the one we used in the *Creeping Down to the Floor* exercise in Lesson 3: No Big Bumps! Ease yourself down.

You're probably thinking, "But in reality a fall happens much faster." That's true, and the next part of the exercise will take that into account.

First, a story. Ira lived in an assisted-living apartment where he could take his meals in the central dining room. His walk had become very slow with very small steps. As he rose from dinner one day and started back along the hall toward his room, he felt a contraction of the light around his eyes. Suddenly he knew he was going to faint and fall. Just before he slipped from consciousness, he remembers saying to himself, from somewhere way back in his mind, "Well, you're going to have to roll with this one." And he did. He actually blacked out and does not remember rolling, but the nurse coming from the other direction says he did a beautiful roll, sinking down to the ground and rolling out to the side. He was not hurt in the least. He had learned to do that roll in an aikido class some twenty-five years before!

Learning to Roll

In the next sequence of exercises you will go back and do the same *Going to the Floor* movements, but you will add something at the end of each. You will slide forward a bit on your hands, turn to lie down on your side, and then roll onto your back.

Too complicated? Not at all. You already know how to do these moves! You learned them in the "Floor Exercises" in Lesson 3. Remember how you got down to your hands and knees from your chair, then lay down on your side and rolled on to your back? Remember bringing your knees up to your chest after *The Table with Two Legs*? These are exactly the same movements, just added on at the end of *Going to the Floor Forward*. So have no fear, you can do it.

EXERCISE 6.4
Rolling Out to the Left

- From a standing position, go the floor to the LEFT, just as you did in the last exercise.
- You will come to the Hip-Sit position.
- Now slide both hands out away from you.
- Lie down on your "long-hand" side. (See figure 6.4a.)

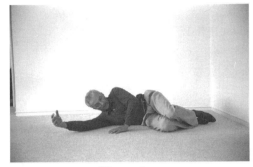

Figure 6.4a

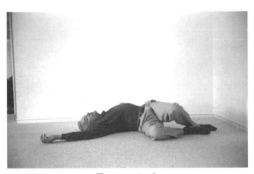

Figure 6.4b

- Roll onto your back. (See figure 6.4b.)
- Bring both your knees up toward your chest. (See figure 6.4c.)
- Then bring your knees back down to the Zero Position.
- Come to rest for a moment.

Roll over onto your knees
- Use your chair to come up to standing.
- Jiggle your hips for a moment to loosen up and settle your balance. Stretch and yawn.
- Come to rest for a moment.

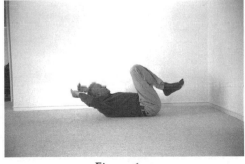

Figure 6.4c

EXERCISE 6.5
Rolling Out to the Right

· From a standing position, go the floor to the RIGHT, just as you did earlier.

· Come to the Hip-Sit position.

· Slide your hands forward and lie down on your "long-hand" side.

· Roll to your back and pull your knees to your chest.

· Bring your knees back to Zero Position, and rest.

EXERCISE 6.6
Rolling Out to the Front

· Start from a standing position.

· Go to the Floor Forward, just as you did before.

· Then, from your hands and knees, SLIDE both hands forward.

· Ease yourself down on your "long-hand" side.

· Roll onto your back.

· Pull your knees up to your chest.

· Then bring your knees back down to the Zero Position.

· Come to rest for a moment.

· Roll over to your side.

· Come to your hands and knees.

· Use your chair to come up to standing.

· Jiggle your hips around for a moment to loosen up and settle your balance.

· Yawn and stretch and pound your chest. Have fun!

· Come to rest for a moment.

Congratulations! You now have all the experience you need. During a fall in real time, you will probably reach the floor with more momentum than in our slow motion practice. When that is the case, you need to *keep going* rather than try to come to an *abrupt stop*. If you come to an abrupt stop, all that momentum makes an *impact* at just one point on your body. That's how you make a bruise on your knee or hip, or strain your wrist or shoulder. When you *keep going*, you spread the impact out over many points on your body without injuring any one of them. You *diffuse* the momentum by rolling onto your back and lifting your knees, instead of *concentrating* the momentum by stopping short.

When you fall, set your hands one short and one long, sit to your hip if you can, slide out onto your side, and roll to your back with your knees up. The rule is simple: **Keep going when you fall, and roll into a ball**.

You will need to do these *Going to the Floor* exercises quite a few times before you begin to feel confident that you can go to the floor safely even in a real fall. Many students have reported that during an unexpected fall, they were surprised that they actually had time to think about their training. They remembered **"Slide! Roll!"** and were able to turn a potentially scary injury into a safe landing.

Of course some students said they only had time to think, "What the heck did he say?" before they landed in an awkward manner. Don't expect a perfect score. Falls can happen suddenly and in strange ways. At those times you have little or no chance of doing much of anything to make the fall easier. All anyone can do is train for the worst and hope for the best.

One sure benefit of these *Going to the Floor* exercises is that you stretch and strengthen the muscles and joints that will take your weight when you *do* fall. Your body will be prepared for the shock, giving you a better chance of coming through a fall with little or no injury. And a second benefit is that, by regular practice, you may reduce your fear of falling sufficiently that you can stay loose and aware during that inevitable fall.

Standing Without Support

So far you have been using your chair as a support when you get back up from the floor. Now you may be ready to try getting back up from the floor without a support. If you have a choice after a fall out in the real world, *always choose using a support over not using one*. After a fall, you may be shakier than you realize. Pride be damned; if there is a lamppost or a car bumper nearby, crawl over to it before you stand up.

But if you don't have a choice, you may need to stand up without support. This exercise will help you practice in case you find yourself on your own.

EXERCISE 6.7
Standing (Without a Support)

- Start on your hands and knees.
- Place both hands at least two feet apart.
- Shift some weight onto your hands.
- Bring one knee up *outside your elbow* and set your foot on the floor.
- Study the triangle made by your two hands and your foot.
- Make that triangle large and more or less equilateral—shift one or both of your hands if you need to.
- Shift your weight forward till your center of gravity is directly over the center of that triangle.
- You will be able to pick up your other leg without much trouble. Do that—pick up your other leg.
- Wave your other leg around a bit to prove how free it is.
- Tip: Don't hold your breath! Breathe naturally with long full tidal breaths. You don't have to be in any kind of hurry. Try yawning in this position (what do you care?) and win a gold star.
- Keep your head down, don't try to lift it at all. Keep your eyes on your triangle instead.

- With your weight still safely over your triangle, put your other foot on the floor.
- Make sure your feet are about two feet apart.
- Put some weight on the foot you just set down.
- Now you are on *four points*, both hands, both feet; you are now a nice big safe quadruped, still breathing naturally, head kept low.
- Shift your weight toward your feet a bit.
- Pick up one hand, wave it around a little. Free, yes?
- Notice the new triangle: one hand and two feet.
- Brace the free hand on your knee.
- Shift all your weight onto your two feet.
- "Pick up the baby," uncurl your spine, and slowly come all the way up to standing.
- Let your head be the very last part to come up.
- Congratulations, you're standing. Bravo, or Brava, as the case may be.

Remember to come up slowly. When you stand up too quickly, you feel a moment of faintness or dizziness. This may only be a brief discomfort, but it can also be a problem; you may risk blacking out for a second and falling. This can happen to anyone, not just to people with Parkinson's. But it is more likely with PD folks because some of the medications you take may lower your blood pressure. Rising too quickly from a prone position can drop the blood out of your head, leading to that unpleasant moment of faintness. So again, come up slowly.

Summary

In this lesson you practiced going to the floor from a standing position.

- You went to the floor to the right, to the left, and forward. You paid attention to every part of the movement, testing the strength of your arms in supporting your weight.

- Then you extended each of your *Going to the Floor* moves by sliding your hands forward, lying out on your side, rolling onto your back, and pulling your knees up toward your chest.

- Finally, you studied the movement strategy for coming to standing "out in the open" without anything to support you.

In this lesson you learned two important pieces of advice:

- Keep going when you fall, and roll into a ball.

- Train for the worst and hope for the best.

If you keep working at it, you'll be ready for anything. Probably nobody with PD can avoid falling, so avoiding injury when you fall is the best goal.

LESSON 7

STANDING STEADY

Now that you have learned to go to the ground from a standing position, you can begin your standing exercises with an additional sense of safety and confidence. If you get into trouble, you can go to the floor with awareness and grace; or at least as much as you can manage.

The first set of standing exercises asks you to free your hip joints by doing hip circles and waist circles. Then you will do a pair of exercises where you place all your weight on one leg while reaching forward with the other. These will help you initiate a step when you find getting started difficult (see the "freezing" discussion in Lesson 10). Then you will stand on one leg while you touch your toe forward, side, back, and then together with the toe of the other foot. You finish with a similar exercise, touching your heel forward instead. These last two exercises will help you make turns (see the "turning" discussion in Lesson 10).

All these exercises are done standing in place with your *eyes steady* on a point across the room. The new idea here will be that your eyes are the second of your three balance systems. When you add **steady with your eyes** to your **postural reflex balance system,** your balance becomes more reliable. Later you will add

hands out from your sides (like a child walking on top of a wall), and you will have a third balancing technique to augment these first two.

Standing on One Leg

You will notice that all of these exercises are done first on the right leg and then on the left. They require you to put your entire weight on each leg in turn. Your overall goal will be to make *each* leg strong and flexible enough to support your entire weight. That will free up your *other* leg to initiate any movement you choose, forward, back, to the side, up and down a stair, into and out of a bathtub or a car. You will also learn to carry your weight evenly on both feet when you stand still. Standing with your weight evenly on both feet may seem obvious enough, but for many people with Parkinson's, it is not obvious at all, as the following story illustrates.

Sister Anne spent seventeen years teaching at the School for the Deaf. She loved her work with all her heart. Languages—spoken and signed—occupied her talented mind throughout her life: she spoke Gaelic, English, Latin, and she could sign American Sign Language "without an accent," which is the highest compliment the deaf community pays a non-deaf signer. She was forced out of her busy teaching career by a quite unusual occupational hazard: carpal tunnel syndrome, from "talking" too much. After a few years spent relocating, retraining for other work, and doing treatments for the carpal tunnel, she developed Parkinson's disease. Those of us who came to love her wondered at these trials. We started off feeling sorry for her, but soon came to feel extremely lucky to have her in our lives.

She was not your typical nun; she came to class dressed in colorful exercise sweats and tennis shoes. But there was something odd about her posture. When she sat on a stool in our classroom, her left hand and wrist would curl tightly in her lap. Her left foot was pulled back a bit, and her left knee tucked itself against her right thigh, like a shy child hiding behind its mother. If you looked more carefully, you could see she tended to rest her weight on the right side of her bottom, tilting slightly to take the weight off the left side. When she stood, she stood with all her weight on her right leg with her left leg lifted at the heel and turned inward.

All of her lively presence had concentrated itself in the right side of her body. Her left side seemed withdrawn, unsure, emptied of energy. Like very many people with the disease, Parkinson's had affected Sister Anne more on one side of her body than the other. The affected side looks and feels weaker, less competent, more hesitant, more tremulous. The foot on that side will often drag a bit. The arm on that side will hold itself close to or even behind the person's body.

Anne had adapted to that loss of ability on her left side by learning to do almost everything with her right. It was as if she had just moved over to the right and vacated her left side, like a person who had closed off the west wing of a house when they could not afford to keep it up.

When we pointed out her right-shifted posture, she was completely unaware of being off center! She could correct the tilt pretty well while she was thinking about it, but as soon as her attention shifted to something else, up she went on her right leg, and the knee would tuck itself away.

Sister Anne had learned to use her right side so well that her left side had actually weakened. Her left wrist had stiffened from disuse. Her left foot was more sensitive than her right when she exercised with the tennis ball under it. When we asked her to shift her weight to the left, she felt some pain in her left leg and hip.

We have all heard the adage, "Use it or lose it." Anne had begun to lose the left side of her body. She needed to challenge her left side to recover strength and flexibility. She needed to work very hard to master these standing-on-one-leg exercises.

Standing Exercises

A word of caution before you begin: You may want to stick with the earlier exercises in this book until you are strong enough to handle the standing exercises safely. Make sure you feel ready. Don't be shy about safety; an ounce of prevention is worth a pound of cure. Do only what you can do safely.

Be careful when you begin these standing exercises. Make special safety arrangements if you tend to fall without warning. Turn your sturdy chair around so the back is toward you. Turn to one side or the other and brace yourself against the chair with one hand while you do the exercises. You may want to stand *between two sturdy chairs* with their backs turned toward you. Better to use more safety than you need.

Test your safety arrangements before you get started on the standing exercises. Hold your hands up in the air a few inches and then grab hold of your chair (or chairs) as if you were about to tumble. Get familiar with how an emergency grab would feel. Don't have any reluctance to make use of your safety supports when you need them.

Now you are ready for the first exercise.

EXERCISE 7.1
Circle Hips

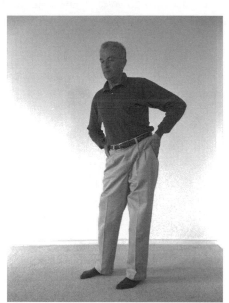

Figure 7.1

- Start from standing.
- Place your feet shoulder width apart, pointing straight ahead.
- Place your hands on your hips.
- Swing your hips in a circle, hula-hoop style. (See figure 7.1.)
- Start with a small, even circle.
- Imagine the circle clearly.
- Try to get your swing as circular as possible.
- Be sure to swing out over your "weak" side.
- Now widen the circle to your limit.
- Make your swing as wide to each side as possible.
- Keep pushing your limits out to the side.
- You will feel the *action* strongest at your hips under your hand. Pay gentle attention to the kinesthesia of your hip joints.
- Make sure you are swinging just as far to the back as you are swinging to the front, and just as far to the right as you are to the left.
- Keep pushing your limits forward and back.
- Do a total of forty circles in each direction. Not necessarily all at once.
- You can change direction anytime you like.

To do the exercises properly, you need to keep your head steady and upright, while your hips swing around under you. Remember the way kids look when they do the hula hoop? Think of the lovely women of Hawaii holding their heads up, proudly and gracefully, as they dance. You don't have to hold your head rigidly in place; just be easy and natural. Don't force things. Try several yawns while you circle your hips.

Steady with Your Eyes

Now I want to add the second part of all these standing exercises: special instructions for how you should use your eyes. Most people, when they begin *Circle Hips*, will gradually expand the circle out farther and make the circling more even. That's all to the good. But people will also stare vacantly at the ground while they do the circles, or their heads will wobble and roll around like drunken sailors. (Sister Anne would gaze absently up to the heavens, which led to some teasing about seeing visions.)

You need to use your eyes to steady yourself. The next exercise will train your eyes to help you to balance.

EXERCISE 7.2
Steady with Your Eyes

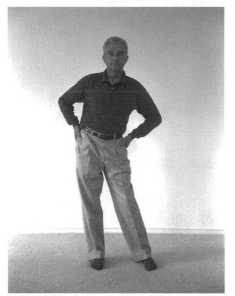

Figure 7.2

- Get your hip circles going.
- Look out at some object at eye level across the room.
- Let's call that object "your spot."
- Let your eyes stay with your spot; keep them steady. (See figure 7.2.)
- Take an interest in what your eyes are seeing (that is to say, don't get glassy-eyed).
- Notice how your moving hips cause the "picture" (what your eyes are seeing) to move a little.
- Try to hold your head still while your hips circle.
- Notice that your eyes can help you hold your head steady.
- Now look at a different spot at eye level.
- Take an interest in the whole field of vision around your new spot.
- Notice how your moving hips cause the "picture" to move a little.
- Again steady what you are seeing by steadying your head.
- Keep your hips circling.
- Change your spot again, steady your head; change again, steady.
- Try looking all the way over to your left.
- Choose a spot, steady your vision, keep your hips circling.
- Do the same thing over to the right.

That's how *Steady with Your Eyes* is done. You can detect your own movement by noticing changes in the movement of your field of vision—your "picture." When your hips move, your head moves; when your head moves, you will see foreground objects change their positon against the background. You will see the periphery of your visual field get wider on one side and get narrower on the other side. *Your brain knows how to use these changes in what you see to keep your whole body steady!* Your brain can't help you if your eyes don't give it the information! So that's your job. You keep your eyes up, and you train yourself to choose a spot, and then keep changing it before your eyes get glassy.

What do I mean by "glassy-eyed"? Well, remember how your eyes get when you are driving on a boring stretch of road? You are not really seeing anything; you're on autopilot. Then suddenly you come back to the present. You wonder, "Who's been driving the car?" And you begin shifting your eyes every few moments to keep your attention in the present. That's what I mean by "Don't get glassy-eyed." Let your eyes move now and then to focus your attention in the present moment.

Your attention should include the whole room you are in during your workout. Attend to your kinesthesia at the center and to your vision at the periphery. You can think of yourself as standing guard, perhaps. Or perhaps you are the lookout on a ship. You could be the lookout in the crow's-nest in an old whaling story; the ship rocking beneath you, your eyes shifting around to each point of the compass. Your attention is steady, receptive; your mind quiet, expectant. At any moment, your glance may catch a sail at the horizon, or a point of land. At any moment, your eyes may catch that plume of spray that means "The whale!"

Now let's continue with your standing exercises.

EXERCISE 7.3
Circle Waist

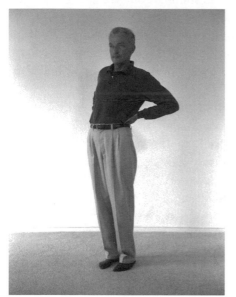

Figure 7.3

- Start from standing.
- Place your feet together, pointing straight ahead.
- Bring your hands around to your lower back.
- Rest your palms against your lower back.
- Feel the muscles of your lower back with your fingers.
- Let your thumbs point toward the front of your waist.
- Swing your waist in a circle. (See figure 7.3.)
- This is a smaller circle than the hip circle.
- Make it a true circle.
- Extend the circle outward toward your limits.
- You will feel most of the *action* under your palms at your waist.
- Choose your spot at eye level across the room.
- Steady your head.
- Keep circling your waist.
- Move your eyes to a different spot, steady your head.
- Change your spot again, steady your head.
- Do these waist circles a total of forty times in each direction.
- Change direction anytime you like. Yawn a lot.

Exercises on One Leg

The following exercise asks you to shift all your weight onto one leg while your other leg moves out in front of you. You want to ask your hip to hold all your weight for just a moment. Then for a moment and a half. Then for two moments. Well, you get the picture.

Sister Anne could stand steady as a rock on her right leg, but, oh, that left leg! "It's as if the poor thing's been asleep for years," she said. The great effort she had to call forth to force herself to trust that leg twisted her face into a grimace. She simply could not be sure of that left leg.

If you are unsure of your balance on one leg, brace yourself by resting your hands lightly on your walker, or on a chair you have placed next to you. You could even have two chairs: one on either side, their backs toward you. Rest your hands *lightly* on the backs of the chairs. You don't want to put any real weight on your hands, because any weight you put on your hands means your leg is not doing all the work.

Hands Away from Hips

If you are steady enough not to need a real chair to brace yourself on, you should set your hands out to each side to brace on imaginary chairs. Remember how children hold their hands out to each side when they walk along on top of a wall? Hands held in this way can help you balance in the same way a long pole helps a tightrope walker balance.

Now you have three balance tools working for you: **postural reflexes** in your foot, **eyes held steady** on an object across the room, and **hands out away from your hips.** Relax, breathe, let yourself feel gravity holding you steady on that one leg, while the other foot is lightly set forward.

EXERCISE 7.4
Toe Touches Forward, Left, and Right

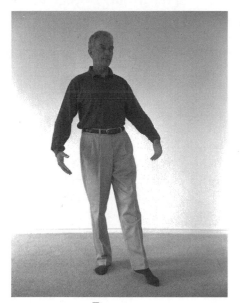

Figure 7.4

- Stand with your feet at shoulder width.
- Hold your hands out away from your hips.
- Imagine a smoldering cigarette on the ground in front of you.
- Shift your weight onto your RIGHT leg.
- Reach your LEFT foot forward and snuff out that smoke with your toe. (See figure 7.4.)
- Bring your LEFT foot back even with the RIGHT.
- Imagine another cigarette on the other side.
- Now shift your weight onto your LEFT leg.
- Reach your RIGHT foot forward, snuff it out.
- Bring your RIGHT foot back even with the LEFT.
- Do this five times on each side.

Notice that your hip rotates in its socket as you crush out that cigarette. If you have done the preceding exercises thoroughly, your hip should feel fairly loose. That means you have relaxed the muscles below and above your hip: below are those long, strong muscles all around your thigh, and above, the short, broad, strong muscles where your spine and pelvis come together. You have also warmed up (literally) the lubricating fluids in your hip socket. Remember how the Tin Man rusted in the rain, and how Dorothy found the oil can and squirted oil into his frozen joints? If you use your imagination, perhaps you can hear your hip sockets creak. Find an imaginary oil can and give your hips a squirt.

EXERCISE 7.5
Heel Touches Forward, Right, and Left

· Stand with your feet at shoulder width.

· Hold your hands out away from your hips.

· Imagine a clump of grass torn up on the golf course. Golfers call that clump a "divot." If you put the divot back and tamp it down, it will live.

· Shift your weight onto your RIGHT leg.

· Bring your LEFT heel forward about 20 degrees from center and tamp that divot down. (See figure 7.5.)

· Tamp all around the edges.

· Bring your LEFT foot back even at shoulder width.

· Now shift your weight onto your LEFT leg.

· Imagine a divot to the other side.

· Bring your RIGHT heel forward about 20 degrees from center and tamp that divot down.

· Bring your RIGHT foot back even.

· Tamp divots five times on each side.

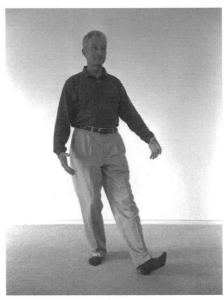

Figure 7.5

Remember that with these two exercises, your weight is all on one foot while your other foot is stuck out there crushing out imaginary cigarettes and repairing that make-believe golf course. Each time you lift your heel to do another crush or tamp, all your weight must be supported by the hip you are standing on. This will strengthen your hip.

EXERCISE 7.6
Toe Touches Front, Out, Side, and Together

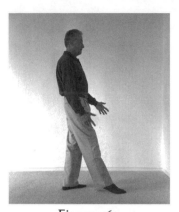

Figure 7.6a

- Stand with feet at shoulder width.
- Hold your hands out away from your hips.
- Shift your weight onto your LEFT leg.
- Bring your RIGHT toe forward, barely touching the ground.
- Eyes steady at eye level.

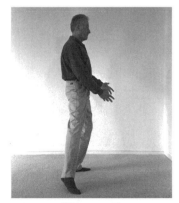

Figure 7.6b

- Pretend you are Fred Astaire or Ginger Rogers for a moment.
- Touch your RIGHT toe to the front, out to the side, to the back, and then together again. (See figures 7.6a—7.6d.)
- Again: front, out, back, together.
- Again: front, out, back, together.
- Again: front, out, back, together.

- Try not to put any weight on the toe that is moving.
- Come to rest for a moment.
- Shift your weight onto your RIGHT leg.
- Bring your LEFT toe forward, eyes steady, dance attitude (remember Fred and Ginger).

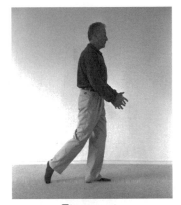

Figure 7.6c

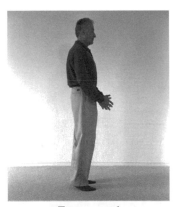

Figure 7.6d

- Touch front, out, back, together.
- Again, three times, front, out, back, together.
- Come to rest for a moment.
- Do *Circle Hips* to loosen up again.

EXERCISE 7.7
Heel Touches Forward 20 Degrees, 45 Degrees, 90 Degrees, and Together

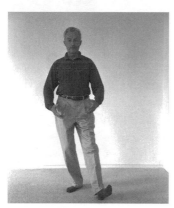

Figure 7.7a

- Stand with feet at shoulder width.
- Hold your hands out away from your hips.
- Shift your weight onto your RIGHT leg.
- Bend your RIGHT knee a little.
- Bring your LEFT heel forward about 20 degrees from center, barely touching the ground. (See figure 7.7a.)

- Eyes steady at eye level.
- Collect yourself, be Fred or Ginger.
- Touch your LEFT heel out at 45 degrees. (See figure 7.7b.)
- Notice that your upper body turns a little.

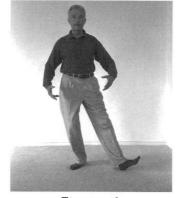

Figure 7.7b

- Touch your LEFT heel to the side, at 90 degrees from center. (See figure 7.7c.)
- Notice that your upper body turns a little more.
- Bring your LEFT foot back beside the RIGHT. (See figure 7.7d.)
- Notice that your upper body turns back to the front.
- Again: touch heel forward 20 degrees, 45 degrees, 90 degrees, together.
- Again, three times.

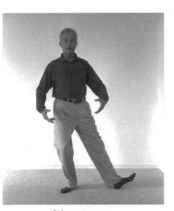

Figure 7.7c

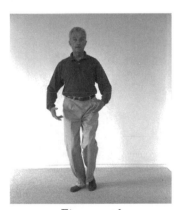

Figure 7.7d

- Come to rest for a moment.
- Shift your weight onto your LEFT leg.
- Bend that LEFT knee a little.
- Bring your RIGHT heel forward about 20 degrees from center, eyes steady, Fred or Ginger.
- Touch your RIGHT heel forward 20 degrees, 45 degrees, 90 degrees, together.
- Again, three times.
- Come to rest for a moment.
- Do *Circle Hips* to loosen up again.

Summary

In this lesson you have begun to improve your balance by challenging it gently and safely:

- Every time you wobble a little on the foot you are standing on, while your other foot is in action—crushing out cigarettes and replacing divots—your wobbly foot and ankle get a bit of exercise.

- Your **postural reflexes** are called into play as your foot and ankle wobble a bit to maintain your balance.

You will get used to making those small adjustments in your foot and ankle that help to maintain your balance.

And you have begun to **use the balance system in your eyes** to help steady you:

- You will get used to keeping your eyes up off the ground.

- You will be using your eyes to steady yourself by focusing on some steady object out there at eye level.

Finally, you have begun to **use your arms and hands as counter weights for balance**:

- You will get used to using your arms and hands held a little away from your sides to serve as your "tightrope walker's balancing pole."

- There will be another series of standing-on-one-leg exercises in Lesson 9.

POWER STANCES

Now you are ready for the second set of standing exercises—the **Power Stances**. These exercises call for you to *create a secure base with feet, legs, and hips*. You will learn *two* power stances, two ways of standing that give you maximum steadiness. Practicing these two stances will add power to your legs and hips.

You will learn to "take a stance" to save yourself from falling; when you begin to lose your balance, you will step into a power stance.

You will also use these power stances to steady yourself before doing something that requires strength or steadiness. These power stances will help you do two things that cause difficulty for many people with Parkinson's: **opening and closing heavy doors,** and **reaching up for something on a high shelf.**

If you are a caregiver, you should learn these power stances, too. If you "take a stance" before pulling your partner up from a chair or out of a bathtub, you will save yourself a lot of sore back muscles.

The Horse

The first stance is called "The Horse" in Tai Chi. When students learn it they are told to imagine a horse between their legs, rather than a barrel. The students train by standing in the horse position facing a wall, their hands forward as if holding the reins. Then they hold the position for thirty minutes! (Don't worry, you are not going to be asked to go to those extremes; three minutes should be enough.)

EXERCISE 8.1
First Power Stance: The Horse

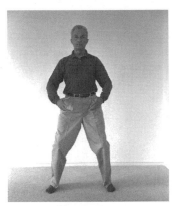

Figure 8.1a

- Start from a standing position.
- Set your feet a bit more than shoulder width apart.
- Point your feet straight ahead, as if your were wearing skis.
- Bend your knees just a little.
- Imagine an upright barrel between your knees.
- Wrap your knees around the barrel to hold it steady.
- Tuck your tail under. (Imagine you are about to sit on a stool.)

- Hold your arms and elbows a little away from your sides, hands forward.
- Hold your hands open wide and curve your fingers, as if you were holding a large ball.
- Rock side to side to adjust your weight evenly at your midpoint.
- Rock forward and back to adjust your weight evenly on both feet.
- Raise your eyes to eye level and look clear across the room.
- Use your eyes to help hold you steady.
- Hold that pose for a full minute. (See figures 8.1a and 8.1b.)
- (Memorize *The Horse*; we'll use it a lot in later exercises.)

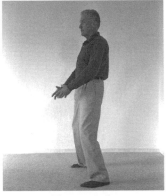

Figure 8.1b

The Horse power stance is one of those universals that apply to almost every sport. What we are calling "The Horse" will be familiar to people who have played soccer. Ernesto pointed out that they might want to call it "The Keeper" or "The Goalie." *The Horse* position allows the goalkeeper to move quickly in any direction to block a shot. A tennis player waiting for service sets up in a very similar posture. A guard in basketball returns to this basic stance when the opponent in front of him has the ball. A skier starting a downhill run comes to this position. Perhaps the most familiar of all is the batting stance in baseball and softball! Put a bat in the hand of a person standing in *The Horse* stance and you'll see what I mean. Do the same with a golf club, and—voilà!—Tiger Woods!

The Bow and Arrow

The second stance, also one of those universal stances, is called "The Bow and Arrow" in Tai Chi. (You have already used this stance when you put one foot forward and one foot back to stand up from a chair.)

EXERCISE 8.2
Second Power Stance: The Bow and Arrow

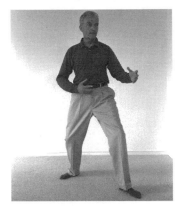

Figure 8.2a

- Start from a standing position.
- Put your LEFT foot forward, RIGHT foot back.
- Set your back foot at about a 70 degree angle to the forward foot. (For the geometrically challenged, just think "more than 45, less than 90 degrees.")
- Bend your knees just a little.
- Open them a little outward.
- Tuck your tail under (remember the stool).
- Set your weight evenly on both feet: not too far forward, not too far back.

- Hold your LEFT hand out over your LEFT foot.
- Hold your RIGHT hand in front of your waist.
- Elbows a little out from your sides.
- Hold your hands open wide, fingers curved, as if holding a large ball.
- Head upright.
- Eyes forward at eye level.
- Hold that pose for a full minute. (See figures 8.2a and 8.2b.)
- (Memorize *The Bow and Arrow*, we'll use it a lot in later exercises.)

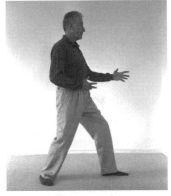

Figure 8.2b

Both of these stances, *The Horse* and *The Bow and Arrow*, will become more effective if you practice them standing still and calm for a *full three minutes*. Start with one minute. Then you should gradually extend your time, a minute at a time, up to three minutes. Don't worry, you won't need to hold still for thirty minutes! But you could set yourself a goal of three minutes during a practice session. A lot can happen in three minutes; you will have time to study and improve many of the fine details of each power stance. You will also engrave these special postures into your physical memory.

Start with only one minute. Extend the time as you feel able. Easy does it.

Think about each of the following corrections while standing in each power stance. It will help to have your helper read these to you, one at a time, while you practice.

- You will have time to become aware of excess tension in your back and learn to release it by gently tucking your tail.

- You will become aware if your balance is too far forward or back on your feet and have time to correct it by shifting your weight back and forth till the weight is evenly distributed.

- You will have time to notice if your eyes have dropped to the ground again, and you will bring them back up to eye level, looking well in front of you. Pay attention to the full panorama of your visual field.

- You will become aware if you are holding your shoulders too high and learn to lower them by reaching down and around with your elbows.

- You will notice if your hands have become slack and droopy, and correct them to the open-wide pulse-warming position you learned in Lesson 1.

- You will find it *necessary* to shift to full tidal breathing, because maintaining this stance for three minutes is not easy! Learn to relax your belly muscles completely as you breathe in; then gently contract your belly muscles as you breathe out. Try to breathe out all your air, completely emptying your lungs. Then relax your belly muscles again for the inhale. Just keep on breathing!

All of these can be summarized into just a few words:

- Knees bent

- Knees open

- Weight even on both feet

- Tail tucked under

- Head up

- Eyes up

- Spine loose

- Both hands open wide and fingers curved

- Breathing full and easy

- Mind peaceful

Moving with the Power Stances

Now for a pair of moving exercises using your first power stance. In both these exercises you will notice your weight shifting from one foot to the other, even though your feet do not lift off the ground at all.

EXERCISE 8.3
Rake In the Goodies

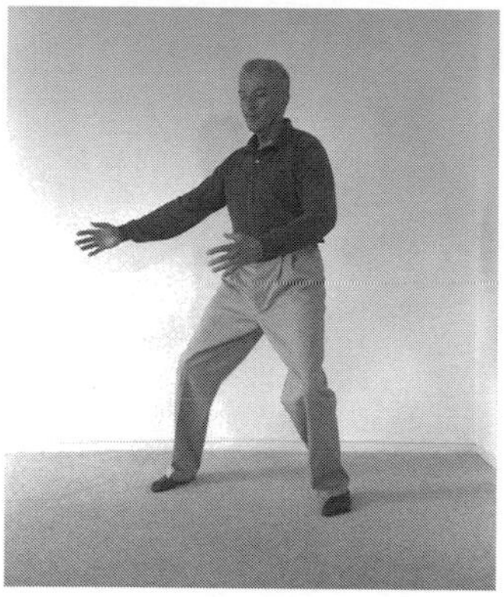

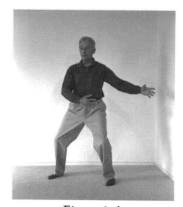

- Come to *The Horse* stance.
- Imagine a high table in front of you.
- Imagine an immense pile of goodies on the table.
- Imagine the barrel between your knees is open.
- Rake in the goodies, hand over hand, into your barrel.
- Reach way forward with your LEFT hand.
- Rake the goodies into the barrel. (See figure 8.3a.)

Figure 8.3a

- Reach way forward with your RIGHT hand.
- Rake the goodies into the barrel. (See figure 8.3b.)
- Hand over hand, hand over hand, twenty times.
- Finish by standing up.
- Shake your legs loose and wiggle your backside to loosen your lower back.
- Do a few *Waist Circles* to loosen up.

Figure 8.3b

EXERCISE 8.4
Throw Goodies to the Crowd

· Come to *The Horse* stance.

· Imagine a barrel full of goodies between your knees.

· Throw goodies to the crowd on both sides of the street.

· Grab a big handful of goodies with your RIGHT hand.

· With a wide sweeping motion, throw the goodies way out to the crowd on the right side of the street. (See figure 8.4a.)

· Grab a big handful of goodies with your LEFT hand.

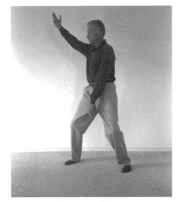

Figure 8.4a

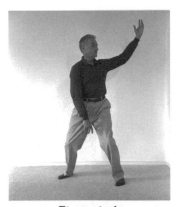

Figure 8.4b

· With a wide sweeping motion, throw the goodies way out to the crowd on the left side of the street. (See figure 8.4b.)

· Hand over hand, throw goodies RIGHT and LEFT, twenty times.

· Finish by standing up.

· Shake your legs loose and wiggle your backside to loosen your lower back.

· Do a few *Waist Circles* to loosen up.

Next comes a pair of moving exercises using your second power stance, *The Bow and Arrow*.

You will be practicing for those moments when you need a sturdy base under you to do something that requires focused power, like pulling open a heavy door or moving a chair.

EXERCISE 8.5
Forward and Back in the Bow and Arrow Stance

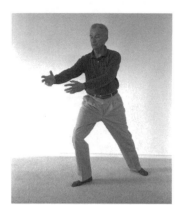

Figure 8.5a

- Come to *The Bow and Arrow* stance, RIGHT foot forward, LEFT foot back.
- Imagine a big log in front of you waist high.
- Imagine a big, old-fashioned, two-handed saw.
- The saw runs parallel to the line through your front foot.
- Grasp the saw handle level with your hips.
- Push the saw forward using mainly your hips first (not your arms!)
- Follow through with your arms.
- Pull the saw backward using mainly your hips first (not your arms!)

- Follow through with your arms.
- Push the saw all the way forward, and stop. (See figure 8.5a.)
- Most of your weight should be on your front leg.
- Make sure your front knee is bent and your body upright.
- Your back foot should still be on the ground, with little or no weight on it.
- Pull the saw all the way backward, and stop. (See figure 8.5b.)
- Most of your weight should be on your back leg.
- Make sure your back knee is bent and your body upright.
- Push forward to the halfway point, and stop.

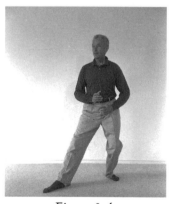

Figure 8.5b

EXERCISE 8.6
Push and Pull a Crosscut Saw

- Go back to sawing the log forward and back as in exercise 8.5.
- Push and pull the saw, twenty times, using your hips first.
- Follow through with your arms with each stroke.

- Finish by standing up.
- Shake your legs loose and wiggle your backside to loosen your lower back.
- Do a few *Waist Circles* to loosen up.

EXERCISE 8.7
Crosscut Saw, Other Foot Forward

- Start from *The Bow and Arrow* stance, this time with your LEFT foot forward and your RIGHT foot back.
- Imagine the log, the saw, and the handle at your hip.
- Saw forward and back, from the hips, twenty times.
- Lead with your hips, follow through with your arms.
- Check to make sure your body stays upright and your knees bent.

- Stop all the way forward, all the way back, and at the center.
- Notice your weight distribution in each position.
- Tuck your tail under! Sit on your buns!
- Finish by standing up.
- Shake loose and do some *Waist Circles*.
- Rest.

Using the Power Stances in Everyday Life

Every person with Parkinson's has a story about doing some difficult physical task that resulted in unexpected consequences. Paul carried a potted azalea to another spot in the garden, bent to put it down, and landed on top of it. Georgia reached up to the second shelf for the big turkey platter, picked it up, and fell backward against the stove. Janet's dog saw a cat, leaped to the right, and pulled Janet to the asphalt. Jules got the groceries out of the front seat, started to walk away, twisted back to shut the car door, and spilled himself and the groceries across the front lawn. "For every action," he said, "there is an equal and opposite reaction, and that proves it."

When you have some work to do that requires some steadiness and some effort, *always set your feet first*. When you walk up to the big glass door at the bank, stand close to the door and set your feet in *Bow and Arrow* before grasping the handle; start your pull with your hips first, then pull with your arm. When you need to close the car door, stand close to the open door, set your feet in *Bow and Arrow* toward the car, take hold of the door handle, then push with your hips first.

Before you had Parkinson's, you used to set your feet *automatically*; now you have to remember to do it *on purpose*. "Power starts in the feet, gathers in the waist, and then pulls or pushes through the shoulders and arms," is the way my Tai Chi teacher, Sifu (Master) Kuo Yien-Ling, explained it. When you practice *Raking in the Goodies, Throwing Goodies to the Crowd*, and *Pushing and Pulling the Crosscut Saw*, think about his words. See if you can find the truth of them in your own movements.

You may remember a movie, *The Karate Kid*, in which an old man trains a boy to box "Okinawa style" by making him polish cars and paint fences, day after day, for weeks. The boy protests that he wants to learn to fight, but the old man firmly and patiently sets him to work again. The old man insists that the boy move the rags while polishing the cars in a particular pattern: "wax on, wax off." He insists that the boy move his paint brush in a sweeping upward motion from the shoulder followed by a similar sweeping-downward motion. Finally the boy blows up and threatens to walk out. The old man tells him to put up his hands and block some punches. The boy says he doesn't know how. But when the old man throws the punches, the boy's arms snap into blocking positions with lighting speed. "See?" says the old man. "Wax on, wax off."

Remember these two power stances. Work them into your daily tasks. When you stand at the counter to prepare dinner, or at the sink to wash dishes, set your feet in *The Horse* stance. Then shift your hips to one side and the other as you pick up a dish over here, wash it in the sink, then put it down over there. Think: "Rake goodies in, throw goodies out." See how that works? When you run the vacuum, stand in *The Bow and Arrow* stance, push the vacuum forward from the hips, pull it back from the hips. Think: "Saw forward, saw back."

Play with these stances during your exercise class. Imagine situations where you might use them. You can step forward into *Bow and Arrow* to the right, then again to *Bow and Arrow* to the left, then right again, then left again; this might be like ice skating. You can step into *The Horse* to the left, then bring your feet together, step left into *The Horse* again; this is like moving sideways between rows of seats at the theater. Play some music and dance with an imaginary partner. You will notice immediately that all the ballroom dances *glide* from the feet first, then move the body from the hips. You don't start dance moves from the shoulders. That gliding motion is the one you want to notice specifically; you will learn to glide your feet into the power stances in Lesson 9, "Balance and Recovery."

Summary

In this lesson you directed your attention to finding two power stances:

- You set your feet apart, bent your knees, tucked your tail, and brought your hands up to the ready. In *The Horse* your feet are set side to side; while in *Bow and Arrow*, one foot is set forward and the other, back.

- You stood still in each power stance for up to three minutes; during that time you studied the internal sense of each stance, correcting your posture to make it strong and memorable.

- You applied *The Horse* stance in a few imaginary work situations in exercises called *Rake in the Goodies* and *Throw Goodies to the Crowds*; while with *The Bow and Arrow* stance you sawed an imaginary log.

- Finally, you imagined everyday situations that might call on you to set your feet in a power stance before you began.

You will use the power stances all through the next lesson, "Balance and Recovery." You will practice gliding quickly into either power stance from every possible direction. That practice will strengthen and train your legs and hips for one of their most important jobs: catching your balance to avoid a fall.

BALANCE AND RECOVERY

In order to practice recovering your balance, you need to practice losing your balance. All the exercises in this lesson involve a **controlled loss of balance** followed by a **planned, graceful recovery**. Think of each exercise as a rehearsal for a fall that almost happens, except that you save yourself every time. Quite the melodrama. And with repeated practice, you'll make recovery look easy.

The Benefits of Balance and Recovery

You have a long list of goals for this practice. First, your goal is to **make each leg *strong* enough to support your entire weight**. The physics here are obvious enough: in order to walk, all your weight must be on one leg while the other is lifted and shifted forward. If you become unsure of the strength of your legs, you may try to keep your weight on both legs as long as possible. If you become too cautious to risk standing on just one leg for very long, you'll begin to take very short steps. These exercises will make you stronger and more confident of your leg strength.

You also want to **make each hip *flexible* enough to allow you to quickly shift your midsection—your center of gravity—to catch your balance**. You want to do that hip-shift while all your weight is supported by that same hip. Every time your free leg changes direction in the air, your standing leg (your "post" leg) shifts at the hip, knee, and ankle to compensate.

You need to practice bringing your free foot, the one you are not standing on, down to the ground quickly and gracefully. **You need to be able to step down in *all* directions**. Hip flexibility makes it possible for you to step forward, to the side, or to the back. You will find a further payoff for your improved hip flexibility in your later work on walking, turning, and overcoming "freezing."

Last, but not least, **you want to learn to step down properly**; that is, you want to step down into one of the two power stances you learned in the last lesson, *The Bow and Arrow* or *The Horse*. A power-stance landing will insure your safety in an emergency.

Landing properly also includes landing without a thump, gracefully and mindfully. You want to **step down to the ground without a sound**. To land "without a sound" you will need to keep your knees bent and flexible; your bent knees serve as your shock absorbers. Learn to step down like an autumn leaf settling to the forest floor. Think of Fred and Ginger, how their feet glide across the floor. Have some fun.

First you need to do a few warm-up exercises. You don't want to try these new and rather challenging exercises by starting cold. Loosen up a bit first; collect your attention; settle down your mind; calm your breathing. Then proceed.

Warm-ups for Balance and Recovery

Warm up by doing four exercises from Lesson 7:

- *Circle Waist*

- *Circle Hips*

- *Toe Touches Forward*

- *Heel Touches Forward*

Standing on One Leg

You may need to take some extra safety precautions for this next series of exercises. Place your sturdy chair beside you with its back toward you, so you can rest your hand lightly there to steady yourself. You may even want a chair on either side, with your hands resting lightly on their backs. You might want to put yourself close to a wall so that, should you fall backward, the wall will catch you. And it may be a good idea to have your helper stand close enough to steady you if you look like you're in trouble. Safety first, then begin the exercises.

Challenge yourself to balance standing on one leg for longer and longer intervals; but keep your safety devices at the ready until you are positive you can do the job unaided. At first you will probably find yourself holding on to the back of the chair with a very tight grip. That's natural enough. After you have gone through the exercise a few times, try loosening your grip until your hand is resting ever so lightly on the back of the chair. Then lift your hand completely off the chair; your hand will be ready to return to the chair if you start to lose your balance. The less you rely on the chair for balance, the more your will be asking of your hips, knees, and ankles to keep you upright. And the more you ask of them, the stronger they will get. Remember, your goal is to make each leg strong enough to hold your entire weight.

A Special Warning for the Foolhardy: Just because you can stand on one leg in exercise class, this does *NOT* mean you should go back to putting on your pants standing up. Don't do it! Forget about it! Sit down to put on your pants! It's one thing to stand on one leg after a series of warm-up exercises and with all your safety devices around you. It's quite another to get your foot tangled up in a pair of pants when you are still half asleep, and you are trying not to wake your partner, and there's all that bedroom furniture and perhaps a hungry cat to contend with. Never take unnecessary risks. People with Parkinson's need to realize they cannot be sure their medications are working well enough—especially in the morning!—to take any chances. It's just not worth it! Remember, *sit down* to put on your pants.

EXERCISE 9.1
Ball Under Foot, Standing

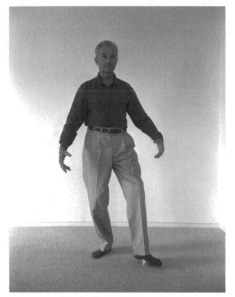

Figure 9.1

- Start from *The Horse* stance.
- Place a tennis ball on the floor about half a foot forward and a little to the LEFT. (It should be in the place your foot will touch when it comes forward and out about 20 degrees.)
- Settle all your weight on your RIGHT leg.
- Rest your hands lightly on your chair supports, if you use them, or
- Hold your arms a little away from your sides.
- Hold your hands open wide, fingers curved.
- Bring your LEFT foot forward and set it lightly on top of the ball. (See figure 9.1.)
- Bring it back right away.
- Bring your LEFT foot forward again and set it lightly on top of the ball.
- Lift your foot off and touch your toe to the RIGHT and then to the LEFT of the ball.
- Set your foot on top of the ball.
- Put some of your weight on the ball, just enough to hurt good.
- Roll the ball a little forward, back, and all around.
- Increase the amount of weight till it hurts *really* good.
- Bring your LEFT foot back to even with the RIGHT.
- Come to rest for a moment.
- Notice the difference in sensations in your two feet.
- Repeat this exercise with the ball under your RIGHT foot.

You will need to work at this *Ball Under Foot* exercise for a while before your feet really learn to love that "hurts good" feeling. You might think of it as a sort of self-administered foot massage, or you may have darker thoughts about self-torture and the bastinado. Just remember, there are many benefits that make *Ball Under Foot* worth enduring:

- **The foot pressing on the ball increases its sensitivity.** Each point on the bottom of the foot becomes more distinct from every other point. You will remember that benefit from the earlier sitting version of *Ball Under Foot*.

- **The leg you are standing on becomes stronger and more balance-responsive.** Strength increases simply by putting your weight on the one leg, the post leg. Balance-response improves as you move the ball foot forward, back, and to the sides, because your post leg—foot, knee, and hip—must adjust to each change in direction.

- **Each time you slip off the ball or start to lose your balance in any direction, you will recover your balance by bringing the ball foot back to the ground.** You may bring it down to the right, to the left, forward or back, but bring it down you must if you want to get balanced on two feet again. Each time you recover your balance in these various ways, your muscles become stronger and more flexible, and your confidence in your ability to catch your balance in an emergency increases.

Balancing on One Leg and Recovering to a Power Stance

Now you are ready for the more challenging work. Go at these exercises slowly and carefully. Do only what you are comfortable with; if you can't bring your knee up to waist level at first, that's fine. Just lift your foot off the ground a couple of inches, brush your thigh instead of your knee, then bring your foot down with as little noise as possible.

Think of each step as separate, but blending into the next, so that all three become one movement. The first few times you do them you will probably do all three quite fast, almost all at once; that's natural, since you will want to recover your balance as quickly as possible. But as you continue your practice, you should gradually *slow down* the three moves; that way, you will *prolong* the moments when you are balanced on one leg. Your helper should also slow down the reading of the instructions to help you slow down the moves. Eventually all three moves will flow together into one movement that is *graceful*, *mindful*, and *complete*.

The slower, the better! The classic sixty-four moves of Tai Chi are practiced at an almost impossible slow-motion pace. This slow pace will build your strength and increase your awareness of kinesthesia. You will notice the little movements inside your hip, knee, and ankle (caused by your postural reflexes) that correct your balance in their subtle way.

EXERCISE 9.2
Step Forward into Bow and Arrow—
Hand Brushes Knee

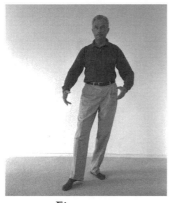

Figure 9.2a

- Start from *The Horse* stance.
- Rest your hand on your chair support, or
- Hold your arms a little away from your sides.
- Set your RIGHT toe forward, stand steady, then

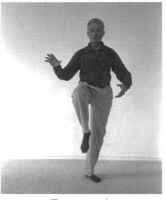

Figure 9.2b

- Knee up,
  - Hand brushes knee,
    - Step *forward* into *The Bow and Arrow* stance. (See figure 9.2a—9.2d.) (Be sure to step down without a sound.)

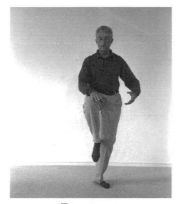

Figure 9.2c

- Come to rest for a moment.
- Repeat to the other side.

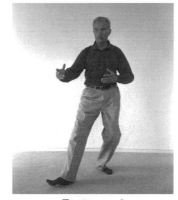

Figure 9.2d

Do this one several times, till it feels easy. Try not to bend down to touch the knee; instead, stand tall, and let the knee come up to you. (Who's the boss, after all?)

Take time to stand steady when you step into *The Bow and Arrow* stance, and correct your posture to get it right. Remember the instructions from the "Power Stances":

- Front foot at 20 degrees

- Knees bent

- Knees open

- Weight even on both feet

- Tail tucked under

- Head up

- Eyes up

- Spine loose

- Front hand over front foot

- Other hand at waist

- Both hands open wide and fingers curved

- Breathing full and easy

- Mind peaceful.

When you are in your power stance, say these instructions over to yourself and make the corrections for each one. Every time you do this, you bring your mind inside your body and focus on the grace of your posture.

Now for a second movement. In this one you turn your knee out a bit, lift your ankle up in front of you as if your were going to pull a burr out of your sock, brush your ankle with the opposite hand, then step forward into your old friend, *The Bow and Arrow* stance. Don't bend down to touch your ankle. Stand tall, and let the ankle come up to your hand.

All the former cautions apply here, too. Use a chair or chairs to either side of you for safety. Don't overdo it. Just bring the ankle up as far as is comfortable, even if that's only five inches, touch your calf with your opposite hand, then step forward as quietly as you can. You'll get better at this one after you've done it several times.

EXERCISE 9.3
Step Forward into Bow and Arrow—
Hand Brushes Ankle

· Start from *The Horse* stance.

· Set your RIGHT heel forward, stand steady, then

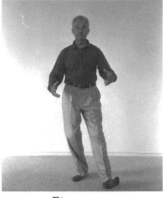

Figure 9.3a

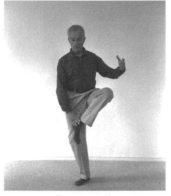

Figure 9.3b

· Ankle up,

  · Hand brushes ankle,

    · Step *forward* into *The Bow and Arrow* stance.
    (See figures 9.3a—9.3c.)
    (Be sure to step down without a sound.)

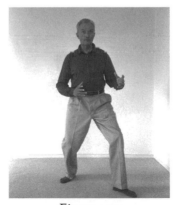

Figure 9.3c

· Come to rest for a moment.

· Repeat to the other side.

Again, let the ankle come up to your hand, don't bend down to touch your ankle. And again, take time to correct your power stance (front foot at 20 degrees; knees bent; weight even on both feet; tail tucked under; head up; eyes up; spine loose; and so forth.)

Practice slowly and calmly; rest when you need to. If you get really tired, just sit down. You can come back to these later—even on another day. *Only you* know when you've done all you can do safely; then you need to decide to take that break.

Now here's a third exercise. This time you'll twist a bit to check the back of your leg, lift your heel up, brush off your heel, then step forward into the good old *Bow and Arrow* stance. Each time you go through it, rest a bit, correct your posture, then get yourself set and give it another go.

EXERCISE 9.4
Step Forward into Bow and Arrow—Hand Brushes Heel

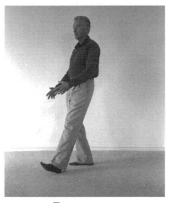

Figure 9.4a

· Start from *The Horse* stance.

· Set your RIGHT heel forward, stand steady, then twist a bit,

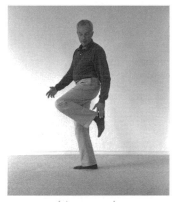

Figure 9.4b

· Heel up,

  · Hand brushes heel,

    · Step *forward* into *The Bow and Arrow* stance. (See figure 9.4a–9.4c.) (Be sure to step down without a sound.)

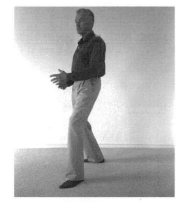

Figure 9.4c

· Come to rest for a moment.

· Repeat to the other side.

You should practice each of these moves till there are no more surprises in them. That may mean two weeks or two months. After a while, you'll notice that you don't have to rush. You'll begin to feel confident that you can lift your knee, ankle, or heel without hurrying. You may even pause for a second or two with your knee up at waist level, like a rooster pauses in mid-strut in the barnyard, then calmly bring your foot down almost to the ground, then glide it forward (like Fred Astaire) into a confident *Bow and Arrow* stance. You may become secure enough to grasp your ankle for a moment instead of just brushing it; then you will release it and glide forward into your stance. You may brush that heel twice—thrice, even five times!— before you float it forward to your stance.

You may also have some near mishaps. Remember to stay calm, ask yourself how the mishap happened, notice what you did to recover your balance. If you can, repeat the same "accident" all over again, so you can learn from it, and take the fear out of it. Congratulate yourself when you succeed in catching your balance.

Rest when you need to. Quit *before* you need to; don't overdo it. Save yourself for another day. If you quit while you're still healthy, "another day" can be as soon as tomorrow.

You can go on to the next exercises after that two weeks or two months of practice that results in a strong sense of confidence.

Recovering to Power Stance in Three Directions

You will now put together the earlier exercises in this lesson in a series that asks you to recover in three directions in succession. You will do each leg-lift three times. The first time you will step *forward* to *The Bow and Arrow*, the second time you will step *sideways* to *The Horse*, the third time you will step *back* into *The Bow and Arrow*. Remember: forward, sideways, back.

The same cautions apply again. You may want to set a chair next to you for emergencies. Bring your knee up only as far as is comfortable. Don't rush. Don't overdo. Rest when you need to. Quit before you have to.

Remember you want to be graceful, mindful, and complete. Throughout all the following exercises, keep these points in mind:

- Keep your eyes focused at eye level.

- Keep your arms a little away from your sides to help with balancing.

- Keep your hands open wide, fingers curved.

- Every leg-lift comes down in one of the power stances.

- Step down without a sound.

- Remember, "forward" is actually about 20 degrees off center; "back" is also about 20 degrees off in the back. If you place your feet in a straight line, as if walking on a tightrope, you diminish your steadiness.

- Don't rush through the moves; hold each power stance for a moment before you go on to the next lift. Correct your stance. Practice completion.

- When you get a little better at the lifts, instead of just brushing the knee, ankle, or heel, hold the lifted pose for a count of two, then three, then four.

In the first section, you'll do your familiar "lift knee, brush, and step" to a power stance. You start from your calm, steady, standing position.

Exercise 9.5
Forward, Sideways, Back—Hand Brushes Knee

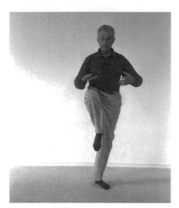

Figure 9.5a

- Start from *The Horse* stance.
- Set your RIGHT toe forward, stand steady, then
- Knee up,
  - Hand brushes knee,
    - Step *forward* into *The Bow and Arrow* stance. (Be sure to step down without a sound.)

- Knee up,
  - Hand brushes knee,
    - Step *sideways* into *The Horse* stance. (See figures 9.5a–9.5c.)

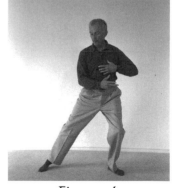

Figure 9.5b

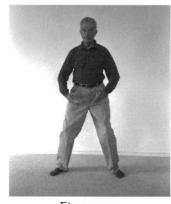

Figure 9.5c

· Knee up,
  · Hand brushes knee,
    · Step *back* into *The Bow and Arrow* stance. (See figures 9.5d and 9.5e.)
· Come to rest for a moment.
· Now set your LEFT toe forward, stand steady, then
· Knee up,
  · Hand brushes knee,
    · Step *forward* into *The Bow and Arrow* stance. (Be sure to step down without a sound.)

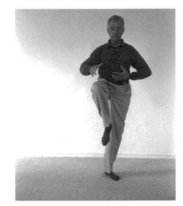

Figure 9.5d

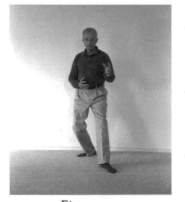

Figure 9.5e

· Knee up,
  · Hand brushes knee,
    · Step *sideways* into *The Horse* stance.
· Knee up,
  · Hand brushes knee,
    · Step *back* into *The Bow and Arrow* stance.
· Come to rest for a moment.

When you step sideways into *The Horse* power stance, remember to correct your stance. The words you need are very similar to the words for *The Bow and Arrow* stance; only foot and hand positions are different.

- Feet apart and pointing forward

- Knees bent and open around a barrel

- Weight even on both feet

- Tail tucked under

- Head up

- Eyes up

- Spine loose

- Both hands forward

- Hands open wide and fingers curved

- Breathing full and easy

- Mind peaceful

In this next section, you'll lift your ankle in front of you and brush it with the opposite hand. Let the ankle come to you, don't bend down to your ankle.

EXERCISE 9.6
Forward, Sideways, Back—Hand Brushes Ankle

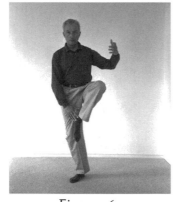

· Start from *The Horse* stance.

· Set your RIGHT heel forward, stand steady, then

· Ankle up,

  · Hand brushes ankle,

    · Step *forward* into *The Bow and Arrow* stance.
    (Be sure to step down without a sound.)

Figure 9.6a

- Ankle up,
  - Hand brushes ankle,
- Step *sideways* into *The Horse* stance. (See figures 9.6a and 9.6b.)
- Ankle up,
  - Hand brushes ankle,
    - Step *back* into *The Bow and Arrow* stance.
      (See figures 9.6c and 9.6d.)
- Come to rest for a moment.
- Now set your LEFT heel forward, stand steady, then
- Ankle up,
  - Hand brushes ankle,
    - Step *forward* into *The Bow and Arrow* stance.
- Ankle up,
  - Hand brushes ankle,
    - Step *sideways* into *The Horse* stance.
- Ankle up,
  - Hand brushes ankle,
    - Step *back* into *The Bow and Arrow* stance.

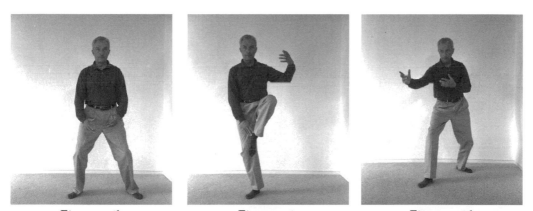

Figure 9.6b   Figure 9.6c   Figure 9.6d

Now for this next exercise, you use the heel-touch pattern you practiced before, and then you make a graceful landing in three different directions.

Exercise 9.7
Forward, Sideways, Back—Hand Brushes Heel

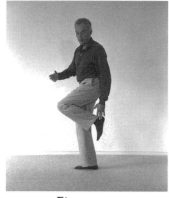

Figure 9.7a

· Start from *The Horse* stance.
· Set your RIGHT heel forward, stand steady, then
· Heel up,
  · Hand brushes heel,
    · Step *forward* into *The Bow and Arrow* stance. (Be sure to step down without a sound.)

· Heel up,
  · Hand brushes heel,
    · Step *sideways* into *The Horse* stance. (See figures 9.7a and 9.7b.)

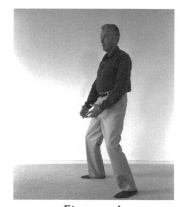

Figure 9.7b

- Heel up,
  - Hand brushes heel,
- Step *back* into *The Bow and Arrow* stance. (See figures 9.7c and 9.7d.)
- Now set your LEFT heel forward, stand steady, then
- Heel up,
  - Hand brushes heel,
    - Step *forward* into *The Bow and Arrow* stance.
- Heel up,
  - Hand brushes heel,
    - Step *sideways* into *The Horse* stance.

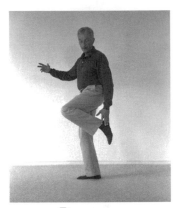

Figure 9.7c

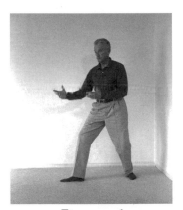

Figure 9.7d

- Heel up,
  - Hand brushes heel,
    - Step *back* into *The Bow and Arrow* stance.
- Come to rest.
- Congratulations!

Summary

In this lesson you did a series of exercises involving a **controlled loss of balance** followed by a **planned, graceful recovery**:

- You arranged safety precautions first, so you could proceed without worrying about getting hurt.

- You practiced placing all your weight on one leg while you lifted the other.

- First you did this with a tennis ball under your foot.

- Then, with one leg lifted, you added a touch to your knee, then to your ankle, and finally to your heel.

- You rounded off each leg-lift by stepping down and gliding into one of the two **power stances**.

- You practiced "coming down without a sound," which encouraged you to soften your landing.

- In the last series, you put together three recovery movements in sequence following each leg-lift: you landed forward, to the side, and to the back, and you did this to both sides.

- You have practiced losing your balance in every direction and strengthened your legs and knees to be ready to catch you if you start to fall.

Let's hope you don't need to recover your balance in an emergency very often. But it's reassuring to know you have practiced for just that eventuality. Remember, you train for the worst and hope for the best.

LESSON 10

WALKING, FREEZING, AND TURNING

Big Jim is the kind of large man who has learned to be extremely polite and helpful to people of less imposing stature—that is to say, most people. He is not used to people offering to help him. One day at the supermarket checkout counter, just as he got his receipt and his change, he discovered that his feet were glued to the floor. For Jim, this was a familiar manifestation of his PD. He could not take a step. Using the edge of the counter for support, he hoisted himself out of the way of the next customer and collected his groceries. And then he did what he had learned to do: he stood there, waiting for his legs to come back on.

The woman behind him eyed him suspiciously as the clerk rang up her groceries. He gave her a small, uncomfortable smile. As she picked up her bags, she could stand it no longer; she looked Jim in the eye and said, "Do you need some help?"

"No, no, I'm okay," said Jim. "Thanks."

She started to leave, but turned back to say, "Can I at least hold the door open for you?"

Not wanting to disappoint such a sympathetic lady, Jim replied, "Yes, that would be nice." Then he thought a moment and added, "When I get there."

Jim was dealing with a moment of **freezing**—a temporary inability to move. Freezing often occurs in doorways or narrow spaces, but sometimes the trigger is unknown. Not all people with Parkinson's experience freezing; but those who do must learn to cope with inconvenient halts in unexpected places. In this chapter you will practice a few techniques to get you moving again when freezing stops you. You will also take a look at two other related problems that often trouble people with Parkinson's: **difficulty making turns** and **festination**—a tendency to take short, accelerating steps when walking.

(Note: These exercises are not meant to be a comprehensive guide to every gait disturbance that can afflict people with Parkinson's disease. Those with serious balance and walking problems should consult a physiotherapist for gait training.)

Working on Walking

You have already done a great deal of work on walking difficulties, though you may not have been aware of it at the time. As a matter of fact, you have been working on walking from the very first exercises in this book. From sensitizing the soles of your feet, to stretching all the muscles surrounding your hips, to reducing your fear of falling, to strengthening your hips to the point where you can bear all your weight on one hip—all these exercises and many others in this program have been preparing you to overcome the difficulties with walking faced by many people with Parkinson's.

In each of your standing exercises, you have practiced shifting your weight from both feet to just one foot and from one foot to the other. If you have practiced regularly, you have already done weight-shifting hundreds of times. You have also set your heel forward and out to the side lots of times; that's the first move in taking a confident step, even during a turn. You've already done all the work; the task now is to *apply* what you've learned to the problems of walking.

This may sound way too obvious, but often the reason you can't pick up your foot is that *you are standing on it!* There is no intention to be facetious here. You may not realize that your weight is resting on the foot you are trying to move. When you experience a freezing moment, most likely you are standing with your weight on both feet. You need to shift all your weight onto just one foot so you can free up the other foot, lift it up, and take that first step. **To start walking, a weight shift is needed.**

That first step is the crucial one. As the proverb has it, "A journey of a thousand miles begins with taking the first step." The solution to getting going is to focus all your mind on taking that first step gracefully and completely. This is another instance of your solution coming by way of GMC—graceful, mindful, and complete. You want to pay attention to the beginning, middle, and end of that one step. Get that first step right, and the rest will come easily, or so we can hope.

The first thing you need to do when you are having trouble trying to get going is to stop. *Stop trying to walk.* Seems paradoxical, doesn't it? But that's exactly what is needed. Remember, "automatic" actions such as those involved in walking sometimes don't work for people with Parkinson's disease. So, when freezing happens, stop trying to walk.

Instead, you are going to concentrate on *taking just the first step*. You will come to rest for a moment. You will collect yourself. You are like an actor pausing in the wings before making an entrance. You'll remember your training, your rehearsal for this moment, and then you'll use what you have learned from your exercises. It's that simple.

The next exercise is the most basic "First Step" exercise. You have done all of this before in earlier lessons; now you are applying it to "freezing" when your feet don't seem to want to move.

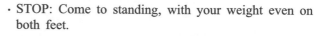

EXERCISE 10.1
Taking the First Step

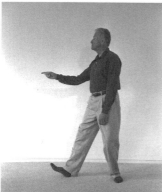

· STOP: Come to standing, with your weight even on both feet.

· Come to rest for a moment. (Come to rest *inside*, too.)

· THINK: "Weight shift is needed." (See figure 10.1a.)

Figure 10.1a

· SHIFT WEIGHT: Shift your weight to one foot; this gets your weight off the foot you want to move. (See figure 10.1b.)

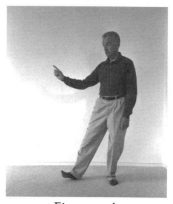

Figure 10.1b

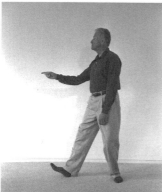

· HEEL FORWARD: Set foot forward at 20 degrees from center, put it down heel first. (See figure 10.1c.)

Figure 10.1c

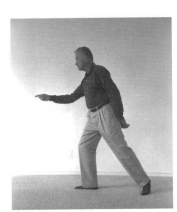

• STEP OUT: Shift your weight forward to your front foot, swing the other foot forward heel first, and walk off, heels first. (See figures 10.1d and 10.1e.)

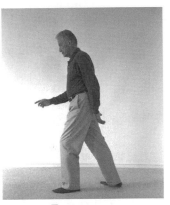

Figure 10.1d

Figure 10.1e

You will want to remember this weight shift technique when you find your feet beginning to freeze, but this may not be so easy; often a person's irritation with their walking difficulty leads to impatience and tightening up. Who wants to remember some dumb motto? You already know that such impatience with yourself will only make things worse. So take the time now to memorize the motto: **Stop; think; shift; heel.**

Memorize that motto! Here is a technique for memorizing that actors use when learning "all those lines" for the parts they play.

- Say the motto out loud eight times right now.

- Then close your eyes and say the motto three times out loud but a little quieter.

- Then keep your eyes closed and say the motto three times moving your mouth as if speaking but without any sound.

- Then without moving your mouth or making any sound, say the words in your mind just to yourself: **Stop; think; shift; heel.**

- Now imagine yourself in a "freezing" moment, weight forward on the balls of both feet. You could exaggerate it a bit in your imagination: see yourself teetering forward, arms waving, a look of desperation on your face.

- Now imagine yourself remembering the motto and *doing* it: **Stop; think; shift; heel.**

- Now open your eyes and say the words out loud.

- That should do it. Now you have almost certainly memorized the words. You will hopefully remember them out there in the real world when you need them.

Taking the First Step—Industrial Grade

Now there may be times when the frozen feeling really threatens to glue your feet to the sidewalk. Your meds may be at a low ebb; you may have been sitting in a car for a long time; you may be tired at the end of your day. You may find that you need a more definite weight shift and a more powerful signal to your other leg that you want it to take the first step.

Again, your cue comes when you discover your feet freezing. You first need to stop trying to walk, and again focus on just that one step. But this time, the first step is actually a half step *back*, followed by a step *forward*, and then walking away.

EXERCISE 10.2
Half Step the Wrong Way First

- STOP: Come to standing, weight even on both feet.
- THINK: "Wrong way first!"
- STEP BACK ONE HALF STEP. This frees up your other foot.
- STEP forward on your free foot, heel first.
- Walk off, heels first.

Difficulty Turning

Wrong Way First also applies to those times when your first step is actually not forward but to one side or to the other, or even a complete 180 degree about-face.

Turning can be a problem for many people with Parkinson's disease. Take Saul Rosenfeld, for example. He usually did the dishes after meals. He found that as he was finishing and starting to turn away to walk across the kitchen, his feet seemed unwilling to move. He would have to catch himself on the edge of the counter to keep from falling.

Many people with Parkinson's disease have difficulty making turns. Again, the essence of your turning problem is most often that your weight is on the foot that you want to pick up and move. Most likely you have begun your turn by turning your head and shoulders around to see where you are going. That's the way almost everybody initiates a turn; for folks without Parkinson's disease there is an automatic weight shift to the opposite foot.

But for a person with Parkinson's disease, turning can be difficult because the "automatic" weight shift to the opposite foot simply does not happen. That leaves your weight on the foot that needs to move next; and there's the problem. Until someone invents antigravity boots that really work, you just won't be able to pick that foot up. You should check this out in action and notice how turning with your head and shoulders first puts your weight on the foot you need to move next.

Of course, you could step *across* that foot you are standing on with the other foot, and that is exactly what many people with Parkinson's do. But stepping across yourself is awkward and can be downright dangerous! You can trip over your other foot quite easily when you try to step across that way. That could lead to a fall. No actor would ever take such a step on stage unless he or she were deliberately showing how awkward and uncoordinated a character is supposed to be. A director's notes to a novice actor would read something like this:

Don't lead with your shoulders! (See figures 10.3a and 10.3b.)

Don't step across your own foot! (See figure 10.3c.)

Shift your weight *away* from where you want to go.

Lead off with your free foot, heel first.

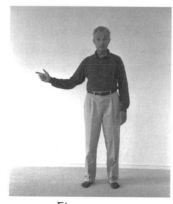
Figure 10.3a

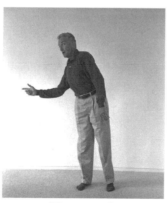
Figure 10.3b

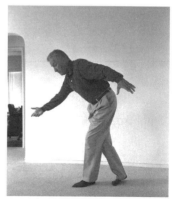
Figure 10.3c

The director would probably underline a few of the words and put two or three exclamation points after each one.

As with *Taking the First Step*, the first thing you need to do is stop. Your cue to stop comes when you feel that stuck-foot-with-twisted-ankle feeling after you have begun to turn. Stop and make your weight even on both feet. Think about what you have practiced. Think: **"Wrong way first; half step; then turn my free foot toward where I want to go."**

Here are the directions for your rehearsal. Do the half step movement over and over again. Practice it in tight corners, between two rows of chairs, and standing pressed against a table or countertop in front of you. Then apply the "wrong way, half step" technique:

EXERCISE 10.3
Turning with a Half Step the Wrong Way

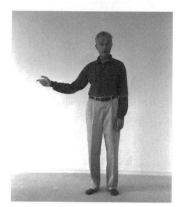

Figure 10.3d

- STOP: Come to standing, weight even on both feet.
- THINK: "Wrong way first!" (See figure 10.3d.)
- STEP A HALF STEP in the direction *opposite* where you want to go. This frees up your other foot. (See figure 10.3e.)
- POINT your free foot in the direction you want to go. (See figure 10.3f.)

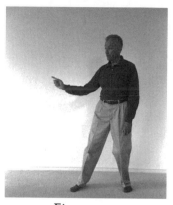

Figure 10.3e

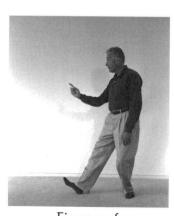

Figure 10.3f

- SET your free foot down heel first.
- (If you want to vary the exercise, set your heel down at 20, 45, and 90 degrees.)
- STEP OUT.
- Walk off, heels first. (See figure 10.3g.)

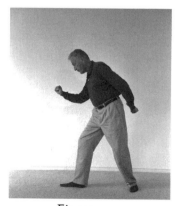

Figure 10.3g

Remember the motto: **Stop; think; half step opposite; point foot and go**.

Stepping sideways to your seat in a theater is a whole series of half-step-wrong-way-whole-step-right-way moves along the row. You should practice this sidestepping maneuver during your exercise workout. Keeping your mind focused on taking *one step at a time* is the key to success.

Mindful Walking

So you succeed in taking that first step, and you set off to trudge the road of happy destiny. As you start to feel confident, your mind turns toward other things, such as where you are going, who will be there, or what you intend to do. Then your steps begin to shorten. "Uh oh!" you say. "Here we go again." Your steps become shorter and shorter till you are up on your toes, almost running in place, and threatening to tip over forward. Sometimes you just manage to stop on your own; sometimes you lose your balance forward. That's when you grab for the wall or a piece of furniture. Then you collect yourself, get that first step right again, and set off again. But the pattern repeats itself: shorter steps, then stuttering steps, and almost falling. It can be very frustrating.

Your tendency to take short, accelerating steps in walking is called **festination**. The source of this common problem may be at that moment *when your mind disengages from the action of walking*. It's a "natural" tendency that almost everybody has: when you get yourself going, you switch to automatic pilot. People ordinarily do not pay much attention to what they are doing, especially if it is routine and familiar. Commuters who listen to books on tape often have no memory at all of actually driving their car along the familiar route. Their minds are completely "elsewhere." But the person with Parkinson's disease cannot rely on the brain's automatic programs. Automatic actions fail the person with Parkinson's at unpredictable moments. That is why we say the person with Parkinson's disease is "condemned to a life of conscious actions."

The trick seems to be to keep at least part of your mind focused on the act of walking. In other words, the trick is **mindfulness**.

Marion uses the magic word "jaunty." When she feels that hesitation that leads to shortened steps, she says to herself, "Jaunty! Jaunty!" She steps out then, heels coming down first, with a little bounce in each step; her arms swing in perfect coordination. This is quite a transformation; it's as if she had never heard of

Parkinson's. And she can keep it up pretty much indefinitely, perhaps because "jaunty" truly suits her personality.

Leo uses a children's chant from his boyhood days. It begins with something like, "Early in the morning you can hear the street cries . . ." and goes on into a seemingly endless variety of street vendor's calls dating back to the turn of the century, all in a marching rhythm. This clever little piece of American history works for him. He sings the first verse as he stands in place marking time, then he steps out on the second stanza. This chant gets him going and keeps him going. Once he gets up to speed he can do two miles and sometimes more along his favorite trail.

Carlos counts cadence and thinks of marching songs from his boot camp days with lyrics that won't bear repeating. Albert starts off saying, "Heel, heel, heel," as his left foot comes forward (that's his more affected side), and then just counts every other step down to the corner. Bridget sings all the verses of "You Are My Sunshine." She says she tried "The Tennessee Waltz" but three-quarter time didn't work for her. (We don't always know when she's just kidding us.) Charley likes waltz time because it makes him "step out a little," left and right, like a skater on the ice, which helps him with his balance. He usually hums something from Vienna, "de de dada, de de dada." Whatever works.

Whatever you choose, work with it till you get that little bounce in your step, and your arms start to swing in **proper coordination**. "Proper coordination" means your opposite arm swings forward when you take a step. (Arm-swing while walking is one of those automatic movements that don't work right with Parkinson's disease.)

- When your LEFT LEG comes forward, your RIGHT ARM comes forward.

- When your RIGHT LEG comes forward, your LEFT ARM comes forward.

You should try this in slow motion to check it out. Exaggerate the arm-swing quite a bit; think of the drum major's strut. Let the arm that is back actually swing back behind you. It may help to hold a handweight or a can of soup in each hand. If you keep at it a while, you'll get that familiar sense of "natural" or "familiar" arm-swinging.

Then try the reverse of proper coordination: deliberately walk with *improper coordination*:

- When your LEFT LEG comes forward, your LEFT ARM comes forward.

- When your RIGHT LEG comes forward, your RIGHT ARM comes forward.

If you are wondering where you've seen this kind of walking before, try exaggerating the stiffness of your arms and legs till your knees don't bend at all and your arms are as stiff as boards. Left arm and leg forward at the same time; right arm and leg forward at the same time. And there you have—the Frankenstein monster! Now you know how Boris Karloff did that trick. The zombies walked that same way in *Night of the Living Dead*.

Don't worry if you get mixed up. All beginning actors get "reverse coordination" when they first pay attention to their own walking: works fine on automatic, but pay attention to how you walk, and your coordination goes to pot. Stick with your practice till it makes sense.

Now it's time to practice walking with your mindfulness cues. First, try to remember one of those songs that you can never forget, the kind that once you start singing it, it just keeps running on and on in your head. Or choose a magic word that describes a graceful gait that suits you: jaunty, dashing, bouyant, chipper, strut, prance, parade, swagger. Choose one or make up your own word.

Second, imagine yourself in a moment of festination. You could even walk along for a few steps and then *demonstrate* how your steps begin to stutter. You can do those festination (or "stutter") steps *on purpose*. Then you can take that moment of hesitation as your cue for your mindful walking exercise.

Exercise 10.4
Mindful Walking

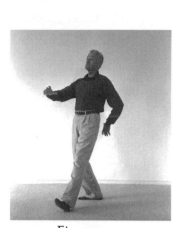

Figure 10.4a

- STOP: Come to rest for a moment.
- THINK: Concentrate on a magic word, song, chant, or cadence to keep part of your mind focused on walking.

- SING a walking song or some ditty you can always remember

    or

- SAY your magic word out loud. Try something upbeat like "Jaunty," "Glide," or "Strut." (See figures 10.4a–10.4c.)

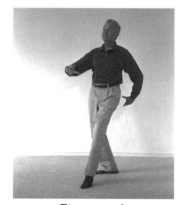

Figure 10.4b

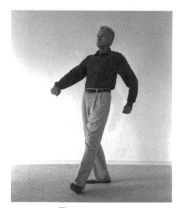

Figure 10.4c

- Sing the song or say the word till you get up to speed.
- Step out, heel first, around the room, or down the hall.
- Let it put a bounce in your step.
- It may even prompt proper arm-swinging.

Estimation

Believe it or not, people with freezing and festination problems often go up and down stairs with no difficulty at all. They may hesitate at doorways, come to an unexpected halt trying to cross a wide-open space, and take stuttering steps upon entering a room, but once they get to the stairs they march right up (or down, as the case may be). It will seem astonishing to strangers who watch a woman with a four-legged walker make her laborious way across the lobby only to reach the stairs, pick up her walker, and climb straight up without a pause.

Another odd observation: people in a freezing moment can sometimes get started by placing a small object (a pencil or a magazine or anything handy) on the floor right in front of their feet; then they step right over the object and continue on their way. An exercise class tried the experiment of placing one-foot strips of blue masking tape across a path all through a large room, down the hall and into the bathroom, and through several doorways. Everyone with gait problems tried walking the path and it worked wonderfully. The class left the tape in place for six months to see if the effect would "wear off" as it became habitual. People sometimes forgot to step onto the path, but when reminded to "use the path" they would step onto it, look down the "blue-tape railroad," and step right out.

The stairs and the blue-tape pathway look similar: they are both a series of regular lines perpendicular to a path. They provide a way of measuring distance, dividing the pathway into a certain number of steps. They seem to establish what one student called a "visual rhythm." Since they both work for most people with Parkinson's disease, that suggests strongly that stairs and taped pathways do something for these people that they are not doing for themselves. What is that something?

These observations suggest an important clue: the problem lies in perception rather than in the legs. In a discussion of reading difficulties experienced by patients with long-standing Parkinson's disease, Roger Duvoisin and Jacob Sage have this to say:

> The problem is not in the eyesight itself. The optical properties of the eye have not changed. The problem is *impaired coordination of the muscles that move the eyeballs from side to side and up and down* [emphasis added]. (From *Parkinson's Disease: A Guide for Patient and Family*, pp. 42–43.)

Since the small muscles around the eye have Parkinson's, too, they sometimes move slowly, festinate, and freeze. Visual perception may indeed be a major factor in your gait disturbances. So what do stairs and taped pathways do for people with Parkinson's disease that they are not doing for themselves? The answer is that they give folks with PD the ability to **measure distance with a quick glance along a path.**

People without Parkinson's disease, just before they start walking, glance out along the path and back, and again from side to side of the path, and automatically calculate the number and length of steps to be taken, which steps to shorten in order to go around an obstacle, and when to begin to twist slightly to go between two obstacles along the path. That automatic glance can happen in a fraction of a second.

People do this without thinking. People make these glances without conscious thought. In a path with many moving objects, say on a crowded sidewalk at the corner of a busy intersection, the number of calculations and recalculations that the eyes and brain must do can be staggering. If you stop to think about it, you'll usually be too slow and get thrown off stride. The automatic calculations of a skilled professional basketball player seem almost beyond belief; we watch the adjustments, the "moves," in slow-motion replay over and over, and we marvel.

"Automatic" doesn't work with Parkinson's. The small muscles around the eye do not make that quick, automatic glance along a path. The brain does not do it's calculations. And the legs don't move.

It is as if the brain will not give the legs *permission* to move until it has made its calculations, and the brain cannot make its calculations until the eyes measure the distances along the path. (It's like a fail-safe program in your ignition that will not let you start your car unless you put it in Park and put your foot on the brake.)

If you can teach yourself to deliberately make these measurements—to consciously look out along a path and back to where you are standing, estimate the number of steps it will take you to get to some spot out there, say your estimate out loud, and then count your steps as you take them to see how close your estimate might be—you will find that you can get moving. You are doing the calculation consciously that the brain does automatically, and that releases the fail-safe and gives the legs permission to move.

EXERCISE 10.5
Estimation Technique

- STOP.
- LOOK out to some point along the way you intend to go.
- ESTIMATE how many steps it will take you to get there.
- STEP off.
- COUNT your steps out loud.
- Keep counting till you get there.
- Stop at the point you had chosen to measure to.
- Look out to some point along the way.
- Estimate, count, stop, and so on.

It doesn't really matter how accurate you are! The point is that you get yourself going with this technique, and that's the real purpose of making the estimate. You don't really have to keep estimating. Just call on this technique when you need it.

Of course, if you want to make a game of it, you could improve your estimates by regular practice. You could keep a sort of mental score of how close you can come.

But you may find yourself cheating a little. Several students who *always* take short little steps found themselves able as the count neared the total of their estimate to take three or four long strides *just to make it come out right!* They were as surprised by their own long steps as anybody else. "Now what's going on here?" their classmates teased them.

Summary

In this chapter you practiced several maneuvers to overcome gait disturbances:

- You learned that a weight shift is needed.

- You practiced **stopping, shifting your weight to one foot**, and **stepping off heel first** with the other foot.

- You learned an "industrial grade" version of the same movement that asks you to take a **half step back** before stepping forward on your free foot.

- You applied the principle of weight shift to **turning** by taking a half-step the "wrong way first," turning your free foot in the direction you want to turn, and then stepping off.

- Finally, you considered the notion that the root of many gait problems may be perception, because the small muscles around the eyes have Parkinson's, too. Since the eyes do not automatically estimate distances and the brain cannot tell the legs that they have permission to move, you need to train yourself to **consciously estimate** how many steps are needed, **say your guess out loud**, then **count off your steps** to see how close you came. You don't have to be very accurate; the estimate itself gets the legs moving, and that's all you need.

Remember: **Heel first, all the time**; unless you are sneaking back into the house at three o'clock in the morning. In that case, tiptoe is probably best.

ADDITIONAL RESOURCES, CONTINUING EDUCATION, AND POLITICAL ACTION

At the first meeting of a new class, some student will inevitably ask, "Do you have Parkinson's?" to which I reply, "No, but I have several other things wrong with me!" My own experience with my share of life's chronic diseases has taught me one thing very clearly, which I now pass on to you: **Everyone with a chronic illness must become an expert on that illness.**

An incurable chronic illness requires that learning about the disease becomes a lifelong task. Parkinson's is incurable and progressive, but it is also the luckiest of the neurological diseases to get, as I heard one neurologist tell a large audience, "because it doesn't kill you." You must become an expert, one day at a time, for whatever time is left you. No particular rush, but you want to get started; focus on each day's problem, learn what you can, prepare yourself for what may come, and just keep on keeping on. Easy does it; but do it.

Further Reading

Here are two excellent books that I recommend to every student. They are both excellent references. Duvoisin is more scientific in his language, while Lieberman uses more ordinary language. Going from one to the other on the same problem can clarify issues from both perspectives. They can also help to answer the questions of relatives who want to know more about it. You can even send them the books to bring them up to speed.

> *Parkinson's Disease: A Guide for Patient and Family* by Roger C. Duvoisin, M.D. and Jacob Sage, M.D. 1996. (Lippincott-Raven, Philadelphia, PA)

> *Parkinson's Disease: The Complete Guide for Patients and Caregivers* by Abraham N. Lieberman, M.D. and Frank L. Williams. 1993. (The Philip Lief Group, Inc., New York)

I suggest that everybody get both books, and that both people in a couple read through both books. Both the caregiver and the person with Parkinson's need to learn all they can. Sometimes the disease can make new learning very difficult or even impossible. Then the spouse or the family member or the caregive rmust become the expert. That sometimes means a reversal of familiar roles: Dr. Dad may need to take over from Dr. Mom, or vice versa.

Keep these books handy, in the same place where you keep daily reference books, cook books, or how-to books. When some new symptom shows up, or when your doctor recommends a new medication, you'll have a ready place to look it up.

Organizations

Here are two national organizations that everybody with Parkinson's should contact. They can supply you with information on your local Parkinson's support groups, they can send you pamphlets and books at very low or sometimes even no cost. They also do important work organizing conferences, supporting research, reporting new information through their newsletters, and advocating for PD with legislatures. They both maintain Websites on the Internet that can link you to many other resources to continue your education and get you involved with other people who are dealing with Parkinson's.

National Parkinson Foundation, Inc.
Bob Hope Parkinson Research Center
1501 N.W. 9th Avenue
Bob Hope Road
Miami, FL 33136-1494
Telephone: (305) 547-6666
Toll Free National: 1-800-327-4545
Fax: (305) 243-4403
Internet E-mail: mailbox@npf.med.miami.edu
World Wide Web: http://www.parkinson.org

The American Parkinson Disease Association, Inc.
1250 Hylan Boulevard, Suite 4B
Staten Island, NY 10305-1946
Telephone: (718) 981-8001
Toll Free National: 1-800-223-2732
Fax: (718) 981-4399
Internet Email: info@apdaparkinson.com
World Wide Web: http://www.apdaparkinson.com/

Research

Researchs have made great leaps in their knowledge about Parkinson's disease during the last twenty-five years. You may be a bit mystified when you first start working your way through a report on a new drug being tested or a new surgical procedure. But soon you will be putting the pieces together, linking one article with another, attending a talk by a pharmacist who finally makes things really clear. When you're up to date, you can be a partner with your physician; when you go in for your appointment you can have questions written out, schedules of medications charted, reports on the occurrence of symptoms with supporting data. Your doctor will be glad of your partnership and will be able to do his job that much better. (If he's not glad, he should be.)

Here's a place where you can get started on learning about Parkinson's disease research. Write them a letter requesting information, check out their Website. They are doing cutting-edge research and they will welcome your inquiry.

The Parkinson's Institute (California)
1170 Morse Ave.
Sunnyvale, CA 94089
Telephone: (408) 734-2800
Toll Free National: 1-800-786-2958
World Wide Web: http://www.parkinsonsinstitute.org/

Political Action

Finally, in your continuing education, you will learn, if you have not learned already, that the way our political world is organized now, each chronic disease must organize politically and lobby for research support, insurance coverage, caregiver relief, home health workers, and the list goes on. You will need to know what is going on in political action groups and find a place where you can do your part to make things work. Here is a good place to start.

Parkinson's Action Network
822 College Avenue, Suite. C
Santa Rosa, CA 95404
Telephone: (707)544-1994
Toll Free National: 1-800-820-4716
Fax: (707)544-2363
Internet E-mail: ParkActNet@AOL.com
World Wide Web: http://pages.prodigy.com/VRGS59A/

The above resources—books, national support groups, a research institute, and a political action organization—should be plenty to get you started on your continuing education.

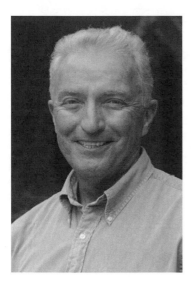

JOHN ARGUE
(Actor, Educator, Writer)

John Argue attended UC Berkeley from 1960-1965, attaining a B.A. in English and later an M.A. in Dramatic Art. During his time at Cal, he won the prestigious Woodrow Wilson Fellow award, the Eisner Prize, and was Regents Fellow in Dramatic Art. After graduation Mr. Argue began teaching acting and theater history at a number of distinguished academic institutions, including UC Berkeley, San Francisco State University, The American Conservatory Theater, and Dell Arte School of Mime & Comedy, among others.

In 1969, he created the Openhand Studio where for sixteen years he taught acting, voice, and improvisation, and wrote, produced, and directed a number of theatrical productions (he won a Drama Critics Award for his play *Anagnorisis*.) In his unique approach to training actors he integrated techniques from the Human Potential Movement, Yoga, Tai Chi Chuan, and Zen meditation. From 1965-1999, Mr. Argue also worked as a professional actor performing in many Bay Area theaters, television commercials, and films. He is a member of Actors' Equity, Screen Actors Guild, and the American Federation of Television and Radio Artists.

In the 1980's, Mr. Argue began working in the field of Drama Therapy, teaching acting in therapeutic settings and working with hospitalized adults and children with disabilities. Recently he has focused on teaching movement and voice classes for people with Parkinson's Disease, developing training regimes that delay and reverse the symptoms of the disease. In 2000, his book entitled *Parkinson's Disease & the Art of Moving*, which trains physical therapists to teach movement to those afflicted with this debilitating disease, was published by New Harbinger Publications. In August 2003, Mr. Argue released a *Video Companion* to his book. He has recently been invited to several cities throughout the US to train teachers in his methods and to encourage the formation of Parkinson's exercise programs.

Mr. Argue presently resides in Oakland, California where he enjoys cooking, gardening, computers, and writing.

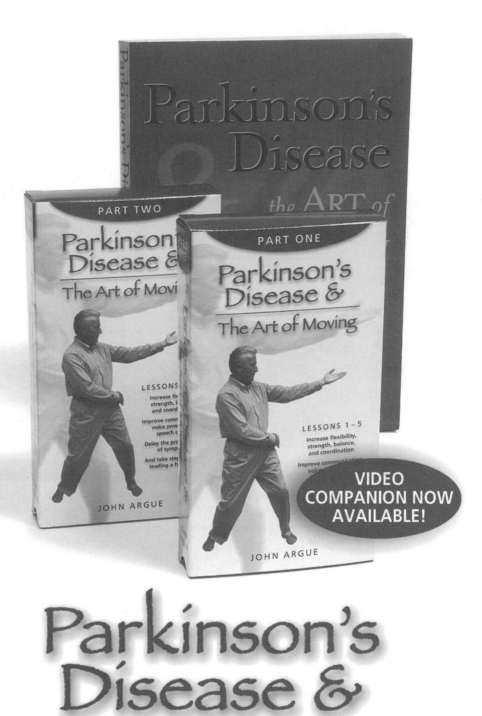

VIDEO
COMPANION NOW
AVAILABLE!

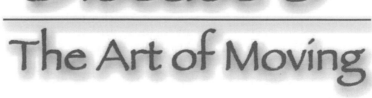

Parkinson's Disease &
The Art of Moving

JOHN ARGUE

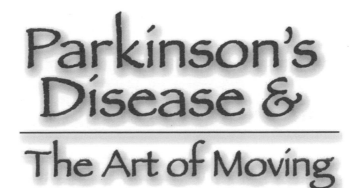

Parkinson's Disease & The Art of Moving

JOHN ARGUE

More New Harbinger Titles

I'LL TAKE CARE OF YOU

Helps family caregivers cope with uncomfortable thoughts and feelings, avoid burnout, access helpful resources, and find ways of meeting their own needs.
Item CARE $12.95

LIVING WELL WITH A HIDDEN DISABILITY

Provides a wealth of resources for healthy living, including advice on navigating the health care system and suggestions for strengthening the body, mind, and soul.
Item HID $15.95

THE CHRONIC PAIN CONTROL WORKBOOK

A team of specialists in all areas of pain management detail the treatment strategies for managing and recovering from chronic pain.
Item PN2 $19.95

WINNING AGAINST RELAPSE

A structured program teaches you how to monitor symptoms and respond to them in a way that reduces or eliminates the possibility of relapse.
Item WIN $14.95

WHAT YOU NEED TO KNOW ABOUT ALZHEIMER'S

Over 150 full-color, illustrated pages explain the underlying biology, provide information about the latest medications and other treatments, and offer practical guidance for coping with the hardships of caring for an Alzheimer's patient.
Item ALZ $15.95

Call toll-free 1-800-748-6273 to order. Have your Visa or Mastercard number ready. Or send a check for the titles you want to New Harbinger Publications, 5674 Shattuck Avenue, Oakland, CA 94609. Include $4.50 for the first book and 75¢ for each additional book to cover shipping and handling. (California residents please include appropriate sales tax.) Allow four to six weeks for delivery.

Prices subject to change without notice.

Some Other
New Harbinger Titles

Eating Mindfully, Item 3503, $13.95

Living with RSDS, Item 3554 $16.95

The Ten Hidden Barriers to Weight Loss, Item 3244 $11.95

The Sjogren's Syndrome Survival Guide, Item 3562 $15.95

Stop Feeling Tired, Item 3139 $14.95

Responsible Drinking, Item 2949 $18.95

The Mitral Valve Prolapse/Dysautonomia Survival Guide, Item 3031 $14.95

Stop Worrying Abour Your Health, Item 285X $14.95

The Vulvodynia Survival Guide, Item 2914 $15.95

The Multifidus Back Pain Solution, Item 2787 $12.95

Move Your Body, Tone Your Mood, Item 2752 $17.95

The Chronic Illness Workbook, Item 2647 $16.95

Coping with Crohn's Disease, Item 2655 $15.95

The Woman's Book of Sleep, Item 2493 $14.95

The Trigger Point Therapy Workbook, Item 2507 $19.95

Fibromyalgia and Chronic Myofascial Pain Syndrome, second edition, Item 2388 $19.95

Kill the Craving, Item 237X $18.95

Rosacea, Item 2248 $13.95

Thinking Pregnant, Item 2302 $13.95

Shy Bladder Syndrome, Item 2272 $13.95

Help for Hairpullers, Item 2329 $13.95

Coping with Chronic Fatigue Syndrome, Item 0199 $13.95

The Stop Smoking Workbook, Item 0377 $17.95

Multiple Chemical Sensitivity, Item 173X $16.95

Breaking the Bonds of Irritable Bowel Syndrome, Item 1888 $14.95

Call **toll free, 1-800-748-6273,** or log on to our online bookstore at **www.newharbinger.com** to order. Have your Visa or Mastercard number ready. Or send a check for the titles you want to New Harbinger Publications, Inc., 5674 Shattuck Ave., Oakland, CA 94609. Include $4.50 for the first book and 75¢ for each additional book, to cover shipping and handling. (California residents please include appropriate sales tax.) Allow two to five weeks for delivery.

Prices subject to change without notice.